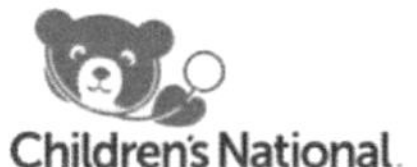

Dear Children's National Colleague,

We've all shared in some great news over the last few weeks: Children's National was named one of the top 10 pediatric hospitals in the country—and our neonatology program was ranked #1 in the nation. I hope you take pride in this extraordinary achievement: you've earned it. But more than any result or ranking, I am most gratified knowing that these awards reflect our world class care for children—care that is possible because of you.

In my 33 years at Children's National, I have been lucky to have truly great mentors, motivating friends, brave patients, and inspiring colleagues. Together, you have shaped my views on pediatric medicine and taught me how to be a better teammate, physician, surgeon, and leader. Most importantly, you've shown me that no competitive edge is as important as the core values we hold dear: our compassion, our commitment, and our connections—to patients and to one another.

That's what truly makes us a top children's hospital.

Over the years, I have also been continually inspired by the brave kids and families who come to us for care. I've learned so much from them about what it takes to help children heal and how to help guide families in their hour of need. I have long felt that these lessons ought to be shared.

That's why I wrote *Healing Children*. My hope is that by sharing stories from my own journey at Children's National, more families can be empowered to get the best possible care for their kids.

The book discusses just a few of the countless patients whose lives have been impacted by the work you do. I am sharing a copy with each of you as a gift of appreciation for your vital role in making these stories possible – and for the courage, kindness, and excellence you bring to our patients each and every day.

No matter what role you play on our team, *everyone* who wears our Children's National badge contributes to our excellence and helps fulfill our mission on behalf of kids everywhere.

Thank you for all you do to help children Grow Up Stronger.

Sincerely,

Kurt Newman, MD
President and CEO

All of my proceeds from Healing Children go to the Pediatric Health Opportunity Fund, a charity supporting research and innovation at Children's National and other research centers.

Healing Children

healing children

A SURGEON'S STORIES FROM THE FRONTIERS OF PEDIATRIC MEDICINE

Kurt Newman, M.D.

VIKING

VIKING
An imprint of Penguin Random House LLC
375 Hudson Street
New York, New York 10014
penguin.com

ISBN 9780525428831 (hardcover)
ISBN 9780698191648 (e-book)

Printed in the United States of America
3 5 7 9 10 8 6 4 2

Set in Ehrhardt MT Std
Designed by Cassandra Garruzzo

To the children, who are my inspiration,

and to the doctors and nurses—and parents—who help heal them.

Contents

PART III:

New Frontiers

Author's Note

The stories in this book are real. They are the stories of children, families, doctors, and nurses, most of whom have come through the doors of Children's National, and meaningfully touched the lives of those who have worked with them. In some cases, I have changed the names or certain identifying details of patients to protect their privacy; in others, all details are unchanged. In one instance, I created a composite character as it seemed to me the only way to fully protect the patient's identity. A desire to help other children and their parents was universally expressed by the families whose stories I have told.

Introduction

Forty years ago I was in my third year at Duke University School of Medicine, working for a future Nobel Prize winner and doing research on receptor molecules in his cardiology lab. I had just drawn a blood sample from an older man at the hospital and taken it back to the lab. I thought I was on to something—using hormones to improve the absorption rates of medication by the body's tissues—and Dr. Robert Lefkowitz, my boss, was pleased with my ideas and results.

I was crouched over the microscope, shifting to analyze the slide, when I reached up and rubbed a spot right below my Adam's apple and found a lump in my neck. I prodded the spot again. I felt a bulging mass, and deep down I knew, though the odds should be in my favor, that I had cancer.

Being a cancer patient at your own medical school is an awkward experience. After a series of tests, Dr. William Peete, a gentlemanly surgeon whose work I had observed during my second year, told me I needed surgery. He was fairly certain I'd be fine, but abruptly I'd found my world turned upside down.

The night of the surgery I checked into the hospital and was so claustrophobic and anxious I could hardly stay put. I managed to persuade the resident, a former classmate, to let me sneak out to play in an intramural basketball game and Cinderella it back by midnight. I stuffed my sneakers and shorts into a backpack and rushed over to the gym, missing warm-ups but taking my regular spot on the bench just as the game began. I played for about two minutes toward the end of the first half, but I was so nervous, I drew a charge call the only time I touched the ball. In the end we lost, and I returned, dejected and even more anxious than before.

I barely slept that night and was sitting straight up the next morning when the orderlies came in to wheel me to the OR—past several of my classmates, who tried to high-five me. One wisecracked about the game the night before. In the OR, to my horror, I realized that the surgical nurse leaning over me was a classmate's girlfriend. Here I was, naked, with Byron's girlfriend looking down into my eyes—that was my last thought before the anesthesia knocked me out.

During those hours and over the coming days, I resolved to become a surgeon. The experience of being fixed and cured by someone else's hands led me immediately to want to cure and fix with my own hands. I still remember what Dr. Peete did in my pre-op exam. He stood in front of me, pulled down his collar, and showed me a scar. He'd had thyroid cancer as a young man, too!

Having experienced surgery while working in a cutting-edge research lab, I began to think that my dream job would combine surgical intervention with scientific investigation. Surgery and science: the present and the future, the hands and the brain. I did not yet realize that this trajectory would entail working with children, but watching a young girl emerge from anesthesia in the recovery room was the first propulsive experience on that path.

I spotted her as I dipped in and out of consciousness, machines beeping, doctors and nurses bustling in the aisle between us. She had short black hair, almost a bowl cut, and must have been around eight years old. Slowly shaking off the anesthesia, I began to register how out of place she was, peering nervously at the machines and all the big people lying on gurneys around her. There wasn't another child in sight. A couple of classmates popped in and started swabbing my mouth with a wet cloth. It felt so dry, I thought my tongue was stuck to my teeth. I wanted to tell them to do the same thing for the girl, but my throat hurt so much, I couldn't get the words out.

Finally one of my friends wandered over and touched her on the shoulder. I felt so relieved—here I was with two buddies boosting my spirits, while she was alone and scared. Even then, long before I could have any role in encouraging policy change to allow parents into recovery rooms, I sensed how wrong it was for this child to be recovering on her own. It wasn't Duke's fault—there probably wasn't a children-only recovery room at any general hospital in the United States at the time—but the image of that girl alone, and the thought of her parents alone somewhere else, stayed with me until I was in a position to do something about it.

In my early years at Children's National, clowns were regular features in the hospital, but an uptight surgeon complained that the clowns had frightened one of his patients, and the administration decided to banish them from the recovery room. Restoring the visitation program was one of my first acts when I became the chief of surgery in 2004. In the intervening years, I treated thousands of children, operated on hundreds, and was regularly amazed by their psychological resilience and bounce-back biology. Kids are genetically programmed to recover from devastating accidents and debilitating conditions. Their biological impulse is to thrive, even in the face of the most daunting conditions.

During my twenty-five years as a pediatric surgeon, I slowly came to grips with the daily risks that children, and their parents, face. Not even a trauma doctor can predict or imagine what trouble a kid will get into. I've extracted a toy soldier from a trachea, an inch-long fish bone from an esophagus, and a shard of an old gym bleacher from a boy's backside. I've helped address terrible burns from ramen noodle spills and tissue damage from snakebites.

Children are made to heal, but they need a medical environment dedicated to creating the conditions in which they can do so. They need, and deserve, more than clowns and child-only recovery rooms. They need specialty centers with doctors, nurses, psychologists, social workers, orderlies, administrators, and maintenance staff devoted to fostering an environment attuned to their unique psychology, biology, and medical conditions. But children's hospitals have struggled to gain a foothold in the lucrative world of American medicine. Adult diseases win more investment; adult doctors are better paid; adult medicine dominates the news cycle. As a society, we prioritize end-of-life and palliative care, while children's medicine is painfully undervalued and underfunded. In the United States there are 35 independent children's hospitals and more than 200 operating as part of a larger integrated health system, but nearly 5,000 hospitals focused primarily on adult care. This in a country with 75 million children under the age of eighteen. My hope is that by the time you finish reading *Healing Children,* you will feel this needs to change.

I am writing this book to share some stunning stories about the children I have treated over the years. Those I write about, with their uncanny fortitude, wit, and wisdom, offer us lessons in how kids can flourish in the face of daunting health challenges if they are treated in a child-first environment.

I have learned a lot in my thirty-plus years in pediatric medicine, and I have also been struck by how often people have turned to me in fear and frustration looking for guidance. Nothing matters more to parents than the well-being of their child. Skillful medical intervention can change the course of a child's entire life, but far too often children are treated by adult specialists who have not been sufficiently trained to address their problems.

As my friends started having kids, I found myself beseeching them to consider using the nearest specialized pediatric center for emergencies, because you are better off going to a pediatric ER if that is an option. Thirty years on I still urge parents to do a dry run to a pediatric ER so they are ready in case of an accident, when minutes can make a difference. If there isn't a pediatric specialty center within range, investigate the varying capabilities of the hospitals that are near you. Do they have specialized pediatric equipment? Do the EMTs have pediatric training? The more pediatric training and specialization—and the more you as a parent know about it—the better the outcome.

Over the years I've followed the entertainment industry's portrayal of my profession with amusement and occasional embarrassment. I've enjoyed the recent run of books by doctors such as Jerome Groopman and Atul Gawande, who have set a high bar for the portrayal of a profession that sooner or later intrigues, inspires, or confounds just about every human being. But there is a large gap in this body of entertainment and literature: the inspiring world of pediatric medicine. I'm writing this book to help fill the gap. The children, parents, doctors, and nurses I've encountered offer the most dramatic and instructive stories of courage and scientific commitment imaginable. My hope is that by reading these stories, parents will discover a new world of medical possibility and will be persuaded to weigh their medical choices alongside other decisions (about schools, sports, and extracurricular activities) into which they put so much time and effort.

When I moved from Boston to Washington as a young surgeon in 1984, I worked for Dr. Judson Randolph—the first full-time pediatric surgeon in the nation's capital. The field has grown since then, and now every year tens of thousands of children are hospitalized, treated, or operated on in specialized pediatric centers. But pediatric surgery and medicine still get short shrift in the overall cultural psyche. Many friends across the country discover the value of specialty centers only when their child ends up at one of them after an unproductive experience at a nonchildren's hospital. Many families I know spend far more time traveling so their children can play soccer than seeking out child-specialized medical care. Some will take the time to rehearse a fire drill at home but never think of planning a trip to the nearest child-focused emergency room in case of an accident. Even my wife and I, both pediatric professionals, once made the simple mistake of not making certain that our health plan covered transport to and care at the closest pediatric specialty center for our children.

Children are biologically and psychologically more suited for exactly the sort of innovative and aggressive treatments that scientific research is producing for adults with such dizzying speed, and I also want to give parents a sense of what makes contemporary pediatric medicine so exciting and transformative. As medical science and technology converge, children's specialty centers are, by virtue of the biological and psychological flexibility of their patients, the perfect spot to implement cutting-edge care. I hope to push pediatric care to a more prominent position in our cultural conversation about medicine, to chronicle for parents the astounding recent advancements in pediatric medicine, and to show them how they can strategically access the best care for their children without having to bankrupt themselves in the process.

This book tracks my own medical and professional journey to illuminate developments in pediatric surgery and medicine over the past forty years. In Part I, I describe how pediatric surgery enchanted me while I was a surgery resident at Brigham and Women's Hospital, a Harvard teaching hospital in Boston, which is perhaps the global center of medicine. This paradox—how I discovered my passion at a place and in a profession that prioritized adult medicine—sets up some of the fundamental themes of this book: the uniqueness of children's biology; the struggle of pediatric medicine to win both esteem and investment; and the critical importance of long-term thinking during every childhood intervention, be it dental surgery or heart surgery, the treatment of a broken arm or of asthma, the selection of a NICU (neonatal intensive care unit) or the approach to overcoming ADD or autism.

In Part II, I introduce my mentor, Dr. Judson Randolph, and his maverick approach to pediatric care. Dr. Randolph embodied the humility and relentless optimism that children crave in their doctors. His style, coupled with his surgical mastery, provided me with a model for my own career—and eventually for the hospital I now run. Dr. Randolph cherished fixing things and solving problems in the short term, with an eye toward a child's long-term life experience.

Next I tell the stories of influential patients and colleagues who transformed my thinking about what pediatric medicine could become if it was treated with the same expansive and creative vision as adult medicine. I realized that if I could combine Dr. Randolph's personal style of humility and optimism with the intellectual, imaginative, and inspirational lessons provided by these patients and peers, I could play my own transformative role in the elevation of pediatric medicine in the United States and in the world.

We doctors often take as much away from our relationships with patients and their parents as they do from us—and what I took away from one relationship helped transform my conception of what a hospital can be and has dramatically improved the lives of many children. Joe Robert, a local businessman whose son I was treating for a complex chest condition, became a sort of secret agent at our hospital—sitting with his son day and night but all the while observing and critiquing us and fantasizing about what we could become. The story of how he helped us take our game to a new level gives an inside look at the future of pediatric care. As I rose through the ranks to become surgeon in chief and then CEO of Children's National, I used the lessons and exhortations from this courageous and inspiring parent to try to establish a radical vision of pediatric care—pain free, aggressive but holistic, and always ready to seek out and embrace innovation.

In Part III, I tell some stories about the type of innovative care—from mental health to orthopedics, from chronic pain management to cancer—that we are developing now. When I became CEO of Children's National in 2011, I decided to prioritize fields like fetal medicine, immunotherapy, behavioral therapy, and pain management because I realized surgery was not the true frontier of pediatric health. It is and always will be part of pediatric care, but as we innovate and push treatments further forward and catch problems earlier, my profession will play a less prominent role in the future of pediatric medicine.

Like several of our fellow children's hospitals, Children's National aspires to a standard of innovative care that kids and parents all over the country should expect to receive and seek to access. The cases I discuss in Part III show how creative childhood treatments are now geared toward transforming the adulthood awaiting each child—not just solving the health issue at hand. This part is a preview of the next frontier in pediatric medicine; it is a call to parents, politicians, and philanthropists to help us realize this bright future. We need to embrace as a society a new vision of pediatric health care that is logical, economical, and compassionate and that takes into account the long arc of a child's life.

I hope that the stories of these amazing children will move and inspire you as they have done me. These kids have been my real teachers, the real drivers of the revolution in pediatric medicine that beckons us so alluringly.

PART I:

Discovering Children

CHAPTER 1:
The Walk Across the Bridge

Entering Ella's room that morning, I had expected to find her resting peacefully with a nasogastric tube sucking bile from her stomach. What I had not expected was to find her parents and grandfather seated in a semicircle around her with their *own* tubes sticking out of their noses and taped to their foreheads.

I was a third-year surgical resident at Brigham and Women's Hospital, making rounds with the senior resident—technically my boss that day—on my first rotation in pediatric surgery at Boston Children's Hospital. Both the Brigham and Boston Children's were teaching hospitals affiliated with Harvard Medical School—many of their doctors taught at Harvard, and Harvard Med School students went there for training and to do their residency. Crossing the bridge between the two hospitals, I had felt the senior resident's mood shift from gruff to decidedly grumpy. Now, as we stood in Ella's room trying to make sense of the scene, I felt he was about to erupt.

He was not the first colleague to show frustration in a pediatric environment. After two years of residency at Brigham and Women's, I had grown accustomed to the regular complaints of my peers as they crossed the bridge to Boston Children's, one of the first and best pediatric specialty centers in the nation. I suppose at some level it was to be expected: they were mimicking an attitude common among the famous doctors who were training us.

Most of my fellow residents were aspiring brain surgeons, cancer researchers, orthopedists, and heart surgeons. They had little time or energy for anxious parents, let alone for the quirks and tantrums of children.

The previous day the senior resident had brusquely informed Ella's parents she would need a nasogastric tube, which we would have to insert through her nose down into her stomach. Her intestine, which we had untwisted in a relatively common but quite invasive surgical procedure, was still not functioning properly, and we needed to relieve it of all stress to give it a chance to heal. Ella's parents had been patiently waiting for weeks to see some progress, and the news of the tube had visibly crushed them. The prolonged hospital stay was taking a toll on their four-year-old daughter, and they worried the tube would further damage her spirits.

The senior resident didn't seem to register their concerns. He silently examined Ella one last time, then wrote out the order for the tube to be inserted.

I wanted to reassure them somehow but couldn't think of what to say or do that wouldn't seem insubordinate.

Ella's parents moved in closer and spoke more emphatically. "She is not ready for this," her father said, his voice not so much stern as weary, almost pleading. "She's been through too much. We have to be able to explain—in her own language—why she needs this."

My colleague looked up and mumbled, "I'm sorry," and then we were off, leaving them with a look of disbelief.

So the following morning when we entered the room, I was struck by the majesty and outrageousness of their gesture.

"We told you we would do whatever it took to make this easier for her," Ella's father said matter-of-factly. Her mother stood up and moved closer. I will never forget the willfulness—the sheer, animallike protectiveness—that she exuded.

The senior resident blushed and didn't even examine the girl before saying, "This is against hospital policy."

I had to do all I could to keep from wincing.

Ella's mother saw that her daughter was registering the tension in our voices and motioned for us to step into the hallway, but the chief resident would not budge. "You are going to have to remove the tubes immediately or we will ask you to leave the hospital," he said.

The grandfather folded his newspaper and frowned. He looked at his granddaughter, then shook his head and closed his eyes.

"Immediately," he repeated, and out he went, before they could respond.

I trailed after him despondently, angry at myself for doing nothing to intervene. I knew he would follow through on his threat, and I could tell the parents understood this. But if it helped the girl, was it really such a problem?

Over the course of my first pediatric surgical rotation, the trips across the bridge had had the opposite effect on me as on most of my colleagues. I loved working at Children's. It felt a bit like going home. I was raised in North Carolina, earned my undergrad degree at the University of North Carolina, and went to Duke medical school, and I was still recovering from a culture shock that had less to do with the infamous rigors of residency at Brigham and Women's than with the gruffness and wear-it-on-your-scrubs ambition of life among hard-chargers up north.

The care and results at the Brigham were excellent, of course, but the coolness and professionalism there, the dispassionate approach to patient interaction, left me wanting. In three short months I had grown to cherish the heightened authenticity I felt every day at Boston Children's. In my first year as a resident, I had made the trip across the bridge a few times during rotations in plastic surgery and neurosurgery, specialties in which there were no separate pediatric departments, but it wasn't until now, in my third year, that I was doing a full rotation in pediatric surgery.

In the end, Ella's parents removed the tubes from their foreheads, and their daughter's intestines began functioning properly soon thereafter. Her digestive system had been given the respite it needed to recover completely. My boss, having done the right thing in the wrong way, departed a year later for a very successful career in adult surgery, and I was left with nagging questions about the system and my future. Why couldn't hospital policies be adjusted to consider the emotional needs of children and their families? Young parents are so desperate to see their children heal. Shouldn't we adjust our ways to address their needs, too? I began to see the bridge connecting the Brigham and Boston Children's as a passage to a different form of medicine, one that accounted not just for the unique psychology and biology of children but also for the concerns of their families.

A few months later I was back on adult rounds in a general male ward at the Brigham that was typically made up of uninsured patients. One night one of my patients, a man we had nicknamed Mr. Pibb, was feeling uncomfortable. He'd had stomach surgery a week before, and the surgeons had placed a nasogastric tube in him, just as they had done with Ella. They wanted his stomach to rest and heal; draining it was key.

The senior resident had directed me to make sure the tube stayed in place all night. Mr. Pibb was notoriously feisty and craved soda pop—hence his nickname, which rhymed with his real name. The painkillers were making him restless, and he was a prime candidate to thrash about and rip his tube out.

The first time the nurse paged me, about midnight, I knew immediately what had happened—the tube had come out. I rushed upstairs and tried to calm Mr. Pibb. Then I gave him all the little extras that I understood to be the hallmarks of a good nasogastric tube insertion. I numbed his nose a little bit to make the placement more comfortable, put the tube on ice to stiffen it a bit so it would be easier to place, and calmly asked him to cooperate with his swallowing as I ran the tube down his throat. Then I taped it in place about as gently as I had ever seen the kindest nurse tape a patient.

An hour and a half later, while I was on my cot catching my first shut-eye of the night, the nurse paged me again. I was by this point, as my mother used to say when I did something wrong, "clearly perturbed." I called upstairs, and the nurse told me that Mr. Pibb had kept thrashing and had pulled the tube out again.

This time I didn't numb his nose or call for ice. I taped the hell out of the tube. I even ordered that he be placed in restraints. Exhaustion and frustration had gotten the better of me, but at least I was certain that he would not be able to dislodge the tube again.

But he did. I had just lain down again when the call came in. A medical student named Robert Sackstein was resting on the cot across the room from me.

"Okay, your turn, Robert," I recall saying. "Nothing like learning on the job." I craved sleep, and having Robert give it a try would buy me a few winks. "But you've got to get them to restrain him completely this time."

The procedure normally takes half an hour with hard cases like Mr. Pibb, so I closed my eyes as Robert got up, and I drifted off before he even closed the door.

But Robert was back ten minutes later. I sat up and asked him what happened.

"What do you mean?" he asked with surprise.

"What happened up there—why are you back so quickly?"

"I put the tube back in and ordered that he be fully restrained," he said.

"That quickly?"

"Well, yes," he said.

"He didn't fight it? He didn't give you a hard time?"

"Well, no," Robert said, obviously trying to get me to shut up so he could get some sleep himself. He turned over, and I suspected he was smiling in the darkness.

"Mr. Pibb did say something to me when I got there," he offered.

"What was that?"

"He said, 'Son, I don't care what you're going to do—just don't call that bald bastard back in here!'"

And with that, Robert broke out laughing. I was, at thirty, already going bald, professional anxiety no doubt expediting genetic destiny. I chuckled and winced not so much at being made fun of as at being found out.

The glaring difference in my experiences of the same procedure on either side of the bridge—and repeated scenarios like it—were starting to make me think that I should go into pediatric medicine. But this was not a field that the best and brightest in Boston's surgical training grounds were encouraged to pursue. Curing cancer and finding solutions for heart disease were the worthy callings for Harvard's most ambitious surgery residents. Pediatric surgery was barely on the radar screen of ambition. I was beginning to feel like a literature student stuck in an engineering class.

CHAPTER 2:
Learning Empathy

During my first year of residency, a famous doctor by the name of Joe Murray was the head of both adult and pediatric plastic surgery. Plastic surgery was one of the few fields that didn't have distinct department heads at Boston Children's and the Brigham. I quickly realized that being assigned to learn from Dr. Murray for two months meant pushing not only my brain beyond its normal capacity but my body, too. I'd hike up and down the "Pike" all day, marveling at Dr. Murray's talents and his stamina. The layout of the place did not make it easy for him to manage his cases.

The Pike was the nickname for the interminable passage that connected all the wards at Brigham and Women's. It began at the emergency room and ended with the bridge to Boston Children's Hospital. On trauma rotations, when you were on call at night, you could be at one end of the Pike stitching a guy who'd been hit in the face with a bottle and then have to race the length of the Pike and across the bridge to treat a child suffering from a dog bite. To fast-walk the length of the Pike was decent preparation for the Boston Marathon, particularly when you had to do it dozens of times a day, as I did when I was following Dr. Murray. He'd resected a small birthmark at Boston Children's, then rush off to do a facial fracture repair at Brigham and Women's. Back then the Pike was worthy of its namesake (the Mass Pike): gritty, cold, and long.

One of the first patients I saw Dr. Murray operate on was a boy who had been badly burned all over his body. Dr. Murray had already performed a series of skin grafts, and the child was progressing marvelously. Like many of his peers, Dr. Murray had gotten hooked on plastic surgery as a military surgeon during World War II. With so many wounded and burned soldiers in need of skin grafts, he had sought to understand the immunology of transplantation. Why was some skin rejected, and what could be done to prevent it? He also became an expert at transplant surgery and was the leader of the surgical team at the Brigham that successfully transplanted the first human kidney in 1954. Decades later, deep into his next passion, plastic surgery, he won the Nobel Prize in Physiology or Medicine his transplant work.

Dr. Murray was reconfiguring this boy's skin and reducing much of his scarring. He was slowly transforming the person he would become, and the boy seemed to know it. Watching them interact lifted my spirits every morning.

After checking in on the boy, we would hustle across the bridge and cruise down the Pike toward the adult plastic surgery ward. Among the first patients I assisted Dr. Murray with at the gloomier end of the Pike was one of the grouchiest, most disheartening patients I have ever encountered. He certainly had reason to be disgruntled. He was in his late fifties and was suffering from a pervasive head, mouth, and neck cancer. The cancer had so eaten into his face and head that Dr. Murray had been forced to do an incredibly complicated restructuring of the man's jaw and cheeks. This was not cosmetic surgery; it was essential for him to maintain some sort of functioning head and neck. In a series of operations, Dr. Murray had replaced the tissue that had been removed with flaps of soft tissue taken from the man's neck, carefully rotating them into place. The work was art and engineering all in one.

Throughout the nearly ten hours of surgery, I stood transfixed as Dr. Murray connected muscle and tissue and flaps. My job was to monitor the patient's blood supply and vitals—such a long surgery could quickly head south—but at times I caught myself losing track as I marveled at his dexterity. But despite my admiration, I questioned his involvement in the case. I was angry at the patient, and this was becoming a troublesome pattern. He had smoked multiple packs of cigarettes a day and had, I believed, inflicted this awful situation on himself. And still he thought he had a right to curse us and accuse us and generally act disrespectfully to the nurses, who were trying to make his life as tolerable as possible.

An impulsive thought kept popping up in my head: *Dr. Murray is wasting his talents and precious time on this grump, when he could be healing kids down the Pike.* I resented my own brain for filling my head with such noxious thoughts and hoped no one could tell what I was silently thinking.

Then one day, at the end of a rotation that included checking in on this man, Dr. Murray pulled me aside and put his hand on my shoulder.

"You know," he said, as if we had been talking about the topic for days, "I think the key to being a good surgeon isn't just mastering the techniques of surgery but caring for the patient. Every patient. To get that outcome that we all want, the care you show after surgery is as important as the success of the surgery itself. It's clear to me that's easier for you with kids, but your obligation of empathy is the same to all your patients."

At first I took his words as a reprimand. My embarrassment faded only slightly as I realized that Dr. Murray had intuited that I was struggling and was encouraging me to follow my heart. I kept walking with him, and he quickly changed the subject to the cases we had seen that day. When we reached his office, I started to walk away, but he motioned for me to come in.

"Here," he said, handing me a nicely bound monograph. I looked down and read the title, *On Caring for the Patient with Cancer.* I had recently heard the lecture itself, given by a world-class cancer surgeon, J. Englebert Dunphy, who had the kind of slightly stilted patrician name I had never heard until arriving in Boston. He was signaling to me with this gift—a monograph not about surgery but about caregiving—that empathy is as important as technical skill.

I looked up at Dr. Murray and saw the expression of gentle care he regularly gave his patients. I took the monograph with a grateful nod and walked back down the hall to Boston Children's. And with that—part admonishment, part encouragement—I felt I had paradoxically been granted the liberty to consider pediatric surgery as a profession. But first I would have to master the caregiving skills that Dr. Murray believed to be so necessary. The man who kept his office in the children's wing and whose body seemed to light up every time he dealt with kids had given me a lesson in bedside manner. From that moment forward, I found myself gravitating toward pediatrics while demanding more of myself in all my work, even when I was taking an exit off the Pike that felt like it might be taking me in the wrong direction.

One last surgery with Dr. Murray, toward the end of my plastic surgery rotation, proved to me that pediatric surgery could be just as thrilling and rewarding as adult surgery was esteemed to be. A five-year-old girl had arrived for surgery to address Crouzon's syndrome, a genetic disorder in which the bones in the skull fuse prematurely, prohibiting its natural growth. The first time I followed Dr. Murray and his team into the girl's room, I steeled myself to face her heartbreaking disfigurement. But the moment we walked through the door, all I could see was a mass of stunning black hair. It was the longest hair I had ever seen on a child, and she obviously took pride in it. It distracted the eye and mind from the physical manifestation of the disease: her eye sockets were sunken and twisted, her cheeks concave, and her jawbone misshapen.

Dr. Murray was partnering on this surgery with the world's leading craniofacial reconstruction surgeon, Dr. Paul Tessier, who was visiting from Paris. I immediately sensed how elegantly Dr. Murray deferred to Dr. Tessier, the man who had revolutionized craniofacial surgery. For all his own accomplishments and fame as a surgeon, he was unabashedly eager to learn from his French colleague.

The sense of collegiality among these two champions of their field left me with an enduring lesson. Here, in front of this proud and hopeful girl, it seemed natural for everyone to pull together and make the well-being of this child our common bond and motivation.

Because of the skills I had developed in my surgery rotations, I was tasked with keeping the girl alive in the pediatric ICU after twelve hours of surgery. The operation was grueling. The surgical team pulled back all the skin on her face, broke just about every bone in her face and many in her skull, stretched her face and jaw into a better fit, and then grafted new bones to hold the structure in place. The anesthesia, loss of blood, and prolonged trauma left me with a daunting task.

The first miracle I witnessed, as I began to monitor the girl in her special recovery room, was how quickly the craniofacial reconstruction achieved its intended effect. Dr. Tessier and his team had developed a series of clay models (today he would have used 3-D printers), and here before me, sleeping deeply, the girl now looked exactly like the model whose face they had sculpted.

The second miracle—at least it seemed so to me at the time—was how quickly the girl recovered. In my few hours in bed the night before the surgery I had tossed and turned, daunted by the prospects of a child recovering from such a massive intervention. Part of me thought it impossible—so much blood, so much risk of immunological rejection, so much trauma in the pushing and pulling of her face. And yet day after day, her vital signs and general responsiveness kept improving. The adult plastic surgery ward, where surgery often inflicts greater trauma than the accident or disease, had accustomed me to the high risks patients underwent not just during surgery but also during recovery. But our young patient was flourishing.

What seemed like a miracle was really just biological logic. Her lungs were healthy—much more so than those of most older patients—her heart was stout, and her immune system had been unaffected by life's toxins, carcinogens, and age. She was the perfect prospect for a successful craniofacial reconstruction. An adult would have been less likely to survive the procedure, and it might not have worked even if he had. The tissues and bones would not have healed as well, and the adult body would have struggled to recover from such a debilitating procedure. Her recovery confirmed for me what many of my colleagues were missing: that pediatric surgery could be more rewarding, more dynamic, and more innovative. The fresh, vigorous biology of young patients made them ideal candidates for aggressive interventions.

CHAPTER 3:
Born to Heal

Pediatric surgery is a young medical specialty in the United States. In the 1970s, when I was in medical school, adult general surgeons still performed most surgery on kids. This was true even at the couple of dozen independent children's hospitals across the country. Duke was a great medical school attached to an extraordinary hospital, but like most hospitals at that time, it lacked a particular dedicated focus on pediatric specialty care. Most pediatric surgeons nationwide were also members of adult surgery departments, and very few nursing units in hospitals were devoted exclusively to pediatric care. During medical school I regularly followed doctors who one minute were treating a seventy-year-old man with coronary artery disease and the next a two-year-old girl who had just had surgery for a ventricular septal defect, otherwise known as a hole in the heart. There were small pediatric wards at Duke Hospital and at many hospitals across the country, of course. But virtually all the surgeons who treated children also performed adult surgery, and most of the anesthesiologists and radiologists cared for both adults and children.

One weekend in my fourth year at Duke, I was trailing a trauma surgeon. A relatively new field at the time, trauma surgery was populated by doctors who had recently been treating soldiers in Vietnam and were now applying their wartime lessons to the accidents and tragedies of daily life at home. Car crashes predominated on weekends, and I was still steeling myself to the sight of mangled bodies and crying children being rushed through the doors of the emergency room.

This particular night the paramedics came racing in with a girl who clearly showed signs of internal bleeding from the trauma she had suffered when a truck hit the car her father was driving. In such a situation, the protocol is to run through a series of rapid checks to determine if the child is in hemorrhagic shock. Is her blood pressure low? How fast is her heart rate? Is she pale due to a loss of blood? Is she lethargic? Hemorrhagic shock results from excessive blood loss—not enough oxygen is carried through the body, especially to vital organs. The heart starts beating faster to compensate. Blood pressure readings can be deceptive as they generally don't drop until the point of crisis. A child will usually sustain a steady blood pressure even longer than an adult, as a child's heart—not yet weakened by heart disease, smoking, stress, and other lifestyle complications—works overtime to pump blood to the body. This resilience can mask internal bleeding.

As the team monitored the various results, I noticed the trauma surgeon gently pressing the girl's abdomen more and more often. Concern filled his face. He must have sensed an expansion in her abdomen—which likely meant her belly was filling up with blood.

Already guessing that her damaged spleen was the source of the suspected hemorrhage, the trauma surgeon quickly decided to take her to surgery to explore her abdomen. He didn't think twice about his decision; it was the protocol in such a case. The exploratory surgery was heavy-duty stuff and entailed its own risks, but saving the girl's life obviously trumped any concerns about additional surgical trauma. I peered over the surgeons' shoulders after they had made a long incision in her belly and saw them nodding to one another as they eyed a laceration of the spleen oozing blood. They quickly decided to remove the girl's spleen entirely.

They achieved their objective: the girl's bleeding stopped. In fact, she recovered with astonishing alacrity. I did not know enough then to wonder—and worry—about the long-term effects of their decision. The spleen is like a huge lymph node, the size of a grapefruit, and it acts as a strainer that traps and filters both white and red blood cells. It then kills the white blood cells that have identified and captured bacteria in the bloodstream. A person can live without a spleen, but we now know that its absence can lead to a vulnerability to infection and, if infection occurs, to rapid sepsis and death.

The strategy of performing a splenectomy had been tried and tested in innumerable adults, and its success, so we thought, meant that it would serve just as well for children. But where is this girl now?

Two years after witnessing that girl's spleen surgery, during my residency in Boston, I discovered an emerging emphasis on fundamental differences between child and adult biology. This awareness would likely have dictated a postponement of the girl's splenectomy—and even of her exploratory surgery—to allow for more prolonged observation. We would have wanted to see if the bleeding would stop and if the spleen would heal itself without surgery. At Boston Children's, pediatric surgeons who had come to understand the uniqueness of children's biology decided that waiting and observing a spleen injury often eliminated the need for an operation. They were guided by the principle that a child's spleen, like many youthful organs, has an ability to heal that is far superior to an adult's. These docs were envisioning the future lives of their pediatric patients—a simple but startling act of imagination that dictated the course and intensity of treatment. Splenectomy should be avoided if possible, for this adult-to-be might need that barrier against infection someday.

This message came home to me one night in my first rotation on pediatric surgery rounds in Boston, when a little boy was rushed into the ER with internal bleeding. This was a confusing time, when seat belts—obviously a major safety advance that was saving thousands of lives—were occasionally themselves the cause of new patterns of injury. The mismatch of adult-size seat belts and children's smaller bodies had led to increased incidences of abdominal injuries in kids.

In my head I was already rehearsing the operation to explore the abdomen and probably remove the spleen. I called the attending surgeon and told him I had to ship a kid with a ruptured spleen to the OR.

"Let me come down and take a look," he said.

I couldn't understand why he wouldn't trust my judgment on what seemed like a straightforward decision to operate.

He arrived and examined the boy thoroughly. "We're gonna wait and watch on this one," he said. "Many of these will heal without surgery. If he does, we've saved his spleen."

The lesson was clear: these surgeons wanted to perform surgery only as a last resort—they didn't want to do what they did best. But the deeper lesson—that they trusted the strength of the boy's vigorous capacity to fix himself—was even more incredible. I learned that children tend to get cracks or lacerations in the spleen rather than a total rupture, which is more common in adults. Kids' organs are more malleable and better able to withstand injury.

Within twelve hours, the boy's signs of internal bleeding—high pulse and low blood pressure, lethargy and slow responsiveness—had subsided. Within forty-eight hours he looked and acted pretty normal. We kept him on bed rest for a week for observation, so as not to trigger any renewed bleeding, but his recovery was impressive and rapid. Unlike an adult, whose biological system needs cajoling and prodding, a child is biologically programmed to heal. Today he is most likely fighting off encroaching bacteria with the best of them, never realizing how lucky he was to have been treated in a children's hospital.

CHAPTER 4:
Making Mistakes

One evening in my pediatric rotation, I was asked to guide a first-year resident through a relatively simple procedure, fixing a child's groin hernia. I'd done it myself a bunch of times, but it was my first time as a teaching surgeon. As I was directing her cut, a gush of yellow fluid spurted out. My chest tightened. I thought the fluid was urine and that we'd slashed the child's bladder by mistake. I wanted to hide my panic from the team, but I had Dr. Tapper paged immediately to get his help.

Many senior docs at Boston Children's seemed to enjoy mentoring, and Dr. David Tapper, a star pediatric surgeon, was like a magnet for many of us. He showed up in an instant and remained totally cool.

"Assess this closely. Don't jump to conclusions just because the fluid was yellow," he said. I was stunned at his calm demeanor.

I probed the bladder and soon realized it was intact. I squeezed the hernia sac slightly, and more yellow fluid leaked out. Dr. Tapper smiled kindly, then winked, to my instant relief. Peritoneal fluid that normally lines the body cavity had collected in the hernia sac. We had not sliced her bladder: we'd done no harm. We finished the procedure, and the infant recovered in no time.

Another surgeon might have been outraged that I'd made such a mistake, or even that I'd interrupted his dinner plans. But Dr. Tapper quickly saw what was going on, how high (or low) the stakes were, and figured out how to proceed so that I'd learn without being humiliated.

Surgeons have a reputation, sometimes merited, for being arrogant and unapproachable. I experienced the best (and worst) of this as a trainee. But Dr. Tapper—Dave, as I later came to know him—symbolized for me the generous attitude that prevailed in pediatric surgery. In this era of collegiality, an implicitly collaborative approach was the rule and not the exception.

Another mentor to many of us who decided to continue with pediatric surgery was Dr. Judah Folkman, the distinguished chief of surgery at Boston Children's. Dr. Folkman taught me how to deal with loss and with the guilt that often follows. During my first two years of residency, I had seen several adults die—of old age, of heart attacks, from gunshot wounds, and from cancer. But until my third year, I had never seen a child die. The realization that they do, and how tragic it is when they do, became a new hurdle to my heeding the pediatric calling.

Toward the end of my second rotation in pediatric surgery, I was treating a teenage boy in the terminal stages of cystic fibrosis, a genetic disease that causes abnormally thick mucus to be produced in the lungs. His lungs were all but shot—scarred from a decade of battling the mucus buildup and infections—and he was on a breathing machine. His family didn't want to give up: we'd gotten his lungs functioning on their own a few times after washing them out, and they were eager for us to try again. This time one lung collapsed, and air got trapped between his lung and rib cage. His medical team decided that he needed a chest tube to help expand his lungs. It fell to me to insert it. Soon after the operation, we realized that his lungs were so feeble, even the tube did not substantially improve his breathing. As he gasped for life over the coming days, it became apparent that the procedure had been in vain.

His overall condition was so precarious that we had actually tipped the scale toward total lung failure. One night he went into cardiac arrest, and I rushed to his room. His family was there, and I instantly sensed their hostility toward me. Everyone seemed to be staring at me, their eyes piercing and unblinking. I had the sense that they felt that my procedure had pushed him over the edge.

He died that night, and for days after that, I lamented the event to a colleague who'd rushed into the room with me. He'd noticed the hostility, too. The situation rattled me like no other. My friend found many small ways to console me, but I couldn't shake my sense of guilt.

Without my knowing it, my friend described my struggle to Dr. Folkman, who was then on the cusp of making one of the most revolutionary cancer discoveries to date: angiogenesis, the science of how tumors co-opt existing blood vessels and force them to provide the nutrition that cancer cells need to grow. One morning at the end of our rounds, Dr. Folkman positioned himself in the hall in such a way as to cut me off from the group.

"I know how you're feeling," he said, cutting straight to the chase. "I know because I've been there many times. You did everything you could for that child, and you're going to save a lot more children in your career. You'll change their lives and give their families the greatest gifts they could receive. Stick to it."

He didn't pat me on the shoulder; he didn't even smile. He darted off to his lab, but he left this massive sense of consolation and courage in his wake.

It wasn't until years later that I discovered one of his own children had died of cystic fibrosis. He knew, both as a doctor and as a parent, how painful it was to lose a child. But he didn't let the shadow of that grief prevent him from doing what he could to help others.

Out of the sixty months of rotations during my residency, I had spent only six at Boston Children's. Had I been given a choice, it would have been much more. I understood the logic of focusing on adult medicine—there were so many more conditions, diseases, and interventions to consider—but the schedule still felt lopsided. Residents today have a chance to acknowledge their passion and interest early and to tailor their course of study more effectively. But when I started, this was far from the case, and I kept looking for confirmation that I was making the right decision.

One night as I lay on the sofa in what must have been my fourth dingy apartment in three years, I tuned in to a new PBS special called *Lifeline*, about the heroes of modern medicine. Each show was devoted to one icon, and in this episode the doctor being profiled was a pediatric surgeon, Dr. Judson Randolph. I sat up when I heard his voice. He was born and raised in Tennessee, and his southern accent both enthralled and unsettled me. Where was he three years earlier when I was feeling like an alien up here?

It wasn't just his slow and steady drawl that captured my attention: in a couple of weeks I was heading down to D.C. for an interview at the hospital whose surgical department he ran, Children's National. It was one of only thirteen pediatric hospitals with a fellowship program in pediatric surgery, offering two years of additional training for surgeons wishing to work with children.

I watched intently as Dr. Randolph spoke to his team about a newborn baby who had just been transferred to the hospital with esophageal atresia, a congenital problem in which the esophagus does not form completely.

"What time was this baby born?" he asked a nurse. "Five hours ago? We've got a good shot at clearing the lungs. Let's get on with it. It's going to be a sweat to get those ends tied together. I don't think we ought to wait any longer. This baby is just too precious to wait."

The camera took us into the operating room, and I was glued to the set as Dr. Randolph described his surgical approach as he painstakingly repaired the baby's esophagus.

"Now we've got to get that upper pouch down here—we have a long way to go, gentlemen," he said, standing over the baby in the harsh light of the OR.

There was silence for about a minute, then Dr. Randolph finally looked up. "Looks good," he said. "I'm satisfied with that."

He took off his gown, removed his rubber surgical gloves, and fired them slingshot style across the room and into the trash can. The camera followed him up to his office, where he kicked back in the chair, put his feet up on his desk, tipped his surgical cap forward, and dialed up the mother to give her a report. Mrs. Vargas was pictured on a split screen in her hospital bed.

With telegenic kindness that George Clooney would have struggled to summon, Dr. Randolph reassured her that her son was doing well.

"Your baby boy looks real good over here," he said. "He looks just fine. I am very pleased, Mrs. Vargas. There are serious days ahead, but we'll give him every support he needs. I'll be talking to you regularly."

I struggled to sleep that night as I wondered what it must be like to work for a man like that in a place exclusively devoted to children. And in the nation's capital, no less. Dr. Randolph's confident, charismatic style assured me that I was headed in the right direction.

CHAPTER 5:
Finding a Mentor

In retrospect, the path I took seems inevitable, but several colleagues and mentors tried to dissuade me from confining myself to what was then seen as a medical backwater. Toward the end of my residency, I started to feel that the manners and pace of my native North Carolina were a metaphor for what I hoped to get out of my medical career. I wanted slower, more intimate, and more homespun interactions with patients. Because of my own cancer scare, I grasped that being a doctor brought with it a much deeper obligation than curing a specific health problem. I was chasing a mirage perhaps, but in an era in which the financial whizzes and insurance companies had not yet taken over medicine, I had a hunch that it would be easier to fulfill my dreams at a pediatric hospital.

When you enter Children's National, you immediately get onto the "people mover"—a long escalator with a slight incline that carries you up from the subterranean parking lot into a bright and colorful atrium. As the contraption slowly took me up to my first real job interview (at age thirty-two—yes, medical studies do stunt your life trajectory a bit), I started to feel that I might finally have hit the jackpot.

The airy atrium—full of giggling children, bustling doctors and nurses, and devoted parents—instantly put me at ease. A band played soft jazz in the corner. Sunlight turned the upper reaches of the atrium a hazy yellow. It felt as if children had been the architects of their own space.

The vitality of the interior came as a relief, for the hospital was what one might politely call a formidable building. Built in the early 1970s in the heavy modernist style that predominated at the time, the dark glass structure abutted the now-abandoned waterworks, a vast field dotted with tiny, decrepit, masonry buildings. It looked like a spaceship that had landed next to a crumbling Civil War battlefield.

As I walked past the cafeteria to the elevator to Dr. Randolph's office, I stopped to breathe in the smell of fried chicken and vegetables. This was long before nutrition was a priority in hospitals, let alone its own department, as it typically is nowadays.

I heard him before I saw him—that magisterial voice and big laugh. Then I spotted the man I had seen on television, huddled with a bunch of nurses. I paused to consider the oddity of the scene. He was huddled with nurses—not docs—and was listening intently to them. I had never seen such a thing in the hierarchical medical world in which I had been training. Docs huddle with docs to hash out tough cases. Nurses simply carried out orders.

When he finished, we sat down on a bench in the hallway, and I prepared for a shift in tone. I had done the standard rehearsals we all do for a job we want: *If he says this, I'll say that.* I had an icebreaker to try to build a bond and two jokes ready for quick dispatch if the moment arose. But all my strategic planning imploded within a couple of minutes. Instead of peppering me with questions, Dr. Randolph did something I was soon to find he rarely does—he talked about himself. He gave me a surprisingly frank assessment of his professional life in Washington.

He told me that when he arrived in 1964, he'd been the first full-time pediatric surgeon in the nation's capital. Children's National was essentially staffed by a group of surgeons who would pass through on given days to operate on kids. The hospital was chartered in 1870 to provide care for the children of the District of Columbia, but for almost a century it would be staffed by surgeons who were essentially moonlighting in pediatric surgery. In the whirlwind two decades Dr. Randolph had been here, he had established one of the country's first fellowship training programs for pediatric surgeons. He had also identified and written about new pediatric conditions and their treatment, essentially claiming for kids their right to have problems once thought exclusive to adults, like gastroesophageal reflux and obesity. He had built a state-of-the-art dedicated burn unit at the hospital and had helped create a new classification system for neuroblastoma, a type of deadly cancer. Most important, he had trained and produced young pediatric surgeons who were spreading out to pediatric hospitals across the country, raising the standard of care and commitment wave by wave.

"You have to understand, a lot of these guys viewed me as a threat," he said, speaking of the general surgeons who dipped in and out of pediatric surgery at the time. "They saw me as the competition, a guy who only took care of babies and children. I don't know if they were worried about losing a portion of their practice, and the money that went with it, or if they were skeptical in general that children deserved their own specialists. Maybe both."

I wondered if he was telling me this as part of his strategy to gauge my devotion to the field. Did he want to elicit shock? Outrage?

Then he startled me out of my suspicions. His face tightened as he described, in painful detail, one of his first "losses," a baby on whom he had performed surgery for a congenital esophageal malformation. The baby had died from complications, and a bunch of adult surgeons on staff at Children's National had tried to pin the tragedy on him. They got so far in their efforts that the hospital undertook a formal investigation into the baby's death. Dr. Randolph was then in his mid-thirties, close to my age, and I began to feel that he might be trying to scare me off.

He'd been determined to clear his name. All it took in the end was to demonstrate that a series of patients with the same diagnosis had died of the same complications—after having been operated on by the same adult general surgeons who had accused him of something between incompetence and negligence. I was enchanted by his defiant tone.

"The infant or small child cannot be treated like a diminutive man or woman," he said, after we visited several of his patients and compared notes about our training up in Boston. "One of my teachers used to say that," he added. "Dr. Gross. You surely know of him?"

Dr. Robert Gross was a legend back at Harvard. He was the father of pediatric heart surgery, among other feats, and I pictured Dr. Randolph following him around Boston Children's as I had Dr. Murray. There was no way not to know Dr. Gross, as he had written the definitive textbooks for pediatric surgical care.

Dr. Randolph didn't tell me I had the job, but as he accompanied me back through the cafeteria, I was wondering what I could do to make sure he did. The atrium was less crowded as I made my way back to the people mover, and the music had stopped. But the place still felt somehow spiritual, and I walked out feeling as if I had a chance to follow a new general leading some sort of a pediatric revolution.

CHAPTER 6:
The Head Coach and His Team

A couple of months later I was sitting in my apartment debating whether to order lobster rolls from my favorite seafood shack at Coolidge Corner or resort to the easy default of a home-cooked "yellow meal" of scrambled eggs and mac and cheese. I had been traveling around the country on a series of interviews, hoping all the while that Dr. Randolph would call me to offer me the job. All the pediatric hospitals I visited were intriguing, but no other doctor matched his charisma. As I took the eggs out of the fridge, the phone rang.

"Dr. Newman," said the familiar voice at the end of the phone. "We've interviewed a dozen impressive candidates, but we'd sure like you to be the fellow here at Children's National. And that guy Cookie Read—tell him he got you the job!"

I nearly dropped the eggs. Dr. Randolph hung up before I could get any details out of him, and he had me laughing as I put down the phone. Cookie Read was a great friend from college, an Episcopal minister who was now based in northern Virginia. One of Dr. Randolph's requirements for the job application had been a letter of recommendation from a nondoctor. I had asked Cookie, and he'd ended his letter with, "Truth be told, I love hanging out with Kurt, and I've written all this simply because I'd sure like to have him nearby."

With Dr. Randolph's blessing, I finished an additional year as chief resident at Brigham and Women's, a position I'd been awarded despite my well-known preference for pediatric surgery. The additional year in adult surgery built my confidence and skills and allowed me to continue to learn from some of the top surgeons in the world. Dr. Randolph, it seemed, was still a believer in the classic American system of training pediatric surgeons. Training in adult surgery was more extensive and more hands on—there were many more adult surgical wards and more adult surgeries to perform. He had told me in my interview that the European model, in which pediatric surgeons specialized much sooner and learned almost exclusively from operations on children, appealed to him but he had bigger battles to fight. I was at peace with my future, and Dr. Murray's advice had stuck. I used the year to focus on cancer surgery and teaching and mentoring surgery residents.

When I finally started at Children's National that hot July 1984, I was quickly struck by how much Dr. Randolph loved sports. He saw life, and his profession, through the prism of a great game. His typical opening conversation with a child usually involved the Washington Redskins or the Atlanta Braves. He was a jock himself and loved to talk basketball technique and strategy with us doctors, too. He equated surgery with athletics and had honed his us-against-them pep talk to rally the surgical staff. He talked about the guts it takes to win tough games and the glory of doing it together.

Sports fan and failed athlete that I was, I lapped it up. I felt an addictive energy every day that summer that I had only really felt playing sports as a kid. Randolph was the coach who knew every detail of each play, the strength and weakness of each player, and who levered the right buttons to motivate and inspire. We had a surgeons' locker room to change into our scrubs, our uniform for the game. There was the presurgery banter, a light jousting to build camaraderie and ease the nerves. And there was the cohesive performance of the team required to make an operation a success—from the seamless passing of instruments to the coordination between the anesthesiologist and the surgeon, and even the exchange of weary high-fives after an eight-hour surgery.

Dr. Randolph had a particular passion for the care of children with burn injuries, and on one of my first rounds with him, he grabbed me and we swooped through the halls toward the burn unit to see a ten-year-old boy named Eddie, who had suffered burns over 70 percent of his body. Dr. Randolph told me that Eddie was recovering from his first skin graft, part of a long, drawn-out process of dressing changes and wound healing. The intense pain of the procedures, the prolonged length of the hospital stay, and the trauma of disfigurement made this a very difficult process both physically and psychologically.

As we headed toward Eddie's room, Dr. Randolph's entourage seemed to be growing by the second. The doctor who had performed the surgery joined us, then two nurses who were caring for Eddie, a social worker, a teacher, and a plastic surgeon. Dr. Randolph abruptly stopped and looked around. I had already observed how he relied on nurses for input and advice, so I supposed that he had a final list of questions for the attending nurse before we went into the nitty-gritty of the next procedure.

"Where's Tom?" he said, his eyes searching the hallway.

I assumed Tom was another social worker—never in my career had I seen such attention paid to the details surrounding a child's case. From around the corner, the mysterious Tom appeared, and I realized he was a doctor.

"Dr. Walsh, what are you thinking about his level of pain today?" Dr. Randolph asked him.

"I'd say seven on the pain scale."

"I'm getting tired of those frowny faces," Dr. Randolph said.

"Jud, we've learned that pain management is critical in cases like this, and if we do it right, we won't have to worry about addiction."

Dr. Randolph thought for a minute, presumably weighing the costs and benefits of using narcotics. "Let's all watch this closely," he said. "Everybody on board?"

"We always do," Dr. Walsh shot back. "We'll reassess daily and adjust pain meds down as soon as we can."

I now understood that Dr. Walsh was a psychiatrist and would have to manage a tricky detoxification procedure if Eddie were to develop a dependency on his pain medication. Dr. Randolph was thinking not just about his patient's physical recovery but about the long-term addictive habits our pain management might burden him with.

After our huddle as we stood by Eddie's bed, I noticed how Dr. Randolph kept making eye contact with Dr. Walsh. When their conversation ended and we all left the room together, the first person he turned to was Dr. Walsh.

"How do you think he is handling the scarring and disfigurement?" he asked.

"He's one of the toughest kids I've encountered," Dr. Walsh said. "'But we need to get these skin grafts done so we can begin reducing the pain meds. If there's any way your team can wrap them up quickly . . ."

Burn victims generally suffer significant scarring, but the accompanying psychological wounds can be just as searing. Dr. Randolph didn't just consider his patients' psychological needs—he prioritized them. He told us again and again that each physical procedure triggered its own psychological consequence, and he wanted both addressed in lockstep. For its time, this holistic approach to healing was startlingly advanced.

It was what most impressed me during my first few months at Children's National. I had never seen such deference to the nonsurgical members of a team. In my experience of adult medicine, preparation for a surgery, its execution, and its measurable result postop were the singular focus of the team. Here I was being introduced to a more expansive definition of success. Each intervention turned into a multifaceted engagement with a child's entire envisioned life, not just her kidney or heart or whatever organ was the immediate issue at hand. How often do we as parents catch ourselves envisioning our children as adults—their jobs, loves, struggles, and pleasures? I think Dr. Randolph performed this exercise with every patient he saw.

An unusual condition that sometimes develops in young people is *pectus excavatum*, a congenital chest disfigurement in which the ribs and sternum grow abnormally. It gives them the appearance of a sunken chest. The condition can surface at birth or manifest itself in puberty. While it is generally not life threatening, it does often lead to the very common adolescent reaction of shame. Dr. Randolph had what I came to realize was a highly developed shame-meter. In situations when parents would bring a boy or girl to us with a sunken chest, I could sense him assessing how the child's self-esteem should play into the decision to operate. He knew that as this child grew into a teenager, their self-esteem could go helter-skelter once confronted with locker rooms, beaches, and dating. But save in rare cases when cardiac and respiratory function were at risk, there had never been any proof that the surgery served any purpose other than cosmetic.

One day a couple brought in their ten-year-old son. I accompanied Dr. Randolph on the consultation. The boy's chest was significantly sunken, and he blushed when he took his shirt off for the exam. The parents seemed flustered, almost ashamed themselves, and it soon emerged that their pediatrician had admonished them not to go see Dr. Randolph, as he was known as an aggressive proponent of surgical intervention in these cases. The pediatrician believed that the risk of surgery was not worth the results. He had told the parents, more or less, that the boy needed to toughen up.

"He said our son needs to accept who he is," they said.

Dr. Randolph winced. He turned to the boy, tousled his hair, and gave him that classic Randolph wink, which always seemed to calm nervous patients. He did a brief examination in which he didn't even look at the boy's chest. He turned to the parents and launched into a series of probing questions on how they envisioned their son's athletic career, dating habits, and social life and asked if they anticipated any family beach vacations while he progressed from, say, age thirteen to twenty-three.

The parents answered honestly, and as they spoke, I could sense the tension going out of their bodies.

Then Dr. Randolph turned to the boy. "You don't like taking your shirt off in public, do you?"

His eyes teared up.

"That's okay, I understand," Dr. Randolph said. "I don't either. You're okay as is, but we're gonna fix you up so all this silly stuff doesn't ever bother you again."

Dr. Randolph had put these parents at ease, letting their own answers bring them to peace of mind. But even more deftly, he had won the boy's trust with understated empathy. He closed with a fact that he loved to tell parents: no one had proven that the surgery actually improved breathing and heart function or athletic ability, but he sure could assemble the data from his case histories to demonstrate a powerful correlation. I would watch him use this personal data to battle several insurance companies into paying for a surgery that he believed was essential. He usually won the battle, and when he didn't, he would find funds from hospital charities to cover the family's costs.

Whether it was burns or scars, caved-in chests or clubfeet, Dr. Randolph taught us not just to analyze the condition in its immediate manifestation but also to consider its long-term effect on the adult-to-be. I wasn't contemplating parenthood myself at this stage—I didn't even have a girlfriend—but I knew that this was the way I would want my own child to be treated.

I was discovering a philosophy of medicine that, while not sentimental, nevertheless embraced sentiment. That was the fundamental difference between my experience of adult general surgery and Randolph's pediatric world. Not that I hadn't seen a heartbroken doctor in the halls of adult hospitals—the death or extreme suffering of a longtime patient could buckle even the steeliest adult surgeon—but most adhere to a clinical methodology that militates against sentiment and relationships. Under Dr. Randolph, the heart accompanied the head from the outset. When later I became a parent myself, I came to appreciate the significance of this approach—and its logic.

CHAPTER 7:
Never Trust the Notes

Surrounded as I was by so many top doctors, the natural thing would have been for me simply to accept the established diagnosis on any case I walked into or inherited. Who was I to question all these impressive brains? That sort of deference was, at the time, typically expected of doctors-in-training. But I soon learned that being a good member of *this* team required a healthy dose of skepticism.

However hard the nurses and nutritionists tried, they could not get baby Jessica to gain weight. She had been hospitalized as a newborn and was now six months old. Soon after birth, she'd started vomiting green bile, and she hadn't stopped since. Her first operation had taken place the day she was born. The surgeons found a blockage in her intestine, caused by a double atresia. In normal intestinal development, one long continuous tube runs from the stomach to the colon. In rare instances, babies will have a gap in the intestine, which is known as an atresia. In Jessica's case, there were two gaps in her bowel, leaving her with a large, abandoned segment of bowel in the middle that had to be reconnected at either end. This was an extremely rare situation, something a surgeon might see once in a lifetime. One gap was somewhat common, but two was almost unheard of.

Jessica's surgeons fixed her intestine by rebuilding it into one continuous tube. They were happy with the technical results of the surgery, but confoundingly, she had made no real progress over the course of six months. A few more exploratory operations were performed, and she was kept alive by nonstop intravenous feeding, but she was still vomiting green. Jessica's doctors had determined that there was no anatomical obstruction. They were baffled. How could her intestine still be getting backed up?

I wasn't directly involved with the case, but it was one of the most frequent topics of conversation among my frustrated surgical colleagues. One day when I was doing the rounds and reviewing cases with Dr. Randolph, he stopped me in the hallway of the neonatal intensive care unit (NICU) and pointed to the baby's room. I glanced over and thought, hopefully, that he had just had an epiphany about the case that was mystifying us all.

"I want you to take a fresh look at that baby girl in the NICU who had the double atresia," he said. "Pretend no one has ever looked at this child. She's had great doctors the whole way through, but sometimes new eyes are the best eyes. Forget all the history. Begin anew."

He shocked me with his instructions. Still room for error with the top docs on his watch, and his own direct involvement?

When I first approached Jessica in her incubator, I felt slightly awkward. What could I bring to the table that hadn't already been thought of? Why me? But I understood my orders.

I spent a few days interviewing everyone who had been involved in the case and reading every note and chart over and over. I visualized what the doctors had been doing as they sewed her intestine together in two places. And I examined Jessica again and again, looking for signs—in her reactions, in her eyes—of some mystery she was hiding from us.

One morning as I stood in front of her almost begging this little creature to reveal her secrets, I suddenly pictured her surgeons' hands unwrapping her intestine. Perhaps, I thought, imagining it all as if in a mental video, the initial bowel surgery hadn't taken into account the simple fact that the intestine, at about the ten-week mark of a pregnancy, exits the fetus, grows, and then rotates as it returns to the abdomen to adhere in its natural alignment. It suddenly occurred to me that the surgical team could have performed the surgery backward. Maybe they had not considered the rotation of the intestine in utero. This would mean that ever since the surgery, the segment of the baby's bowel between the two atresia repairs had been functioning in reverse. It seemed unlikely, but was at least a plausible explanation.

To test this theory, Dr. Bruce Markle, one of our radiologists, suggested that we insert contrast as an enema through Jessica's rectum. So we gathered around and watched, in real time, as the contrast reached the problematic segment of her intestine. Amazingly, it propelled the contrast up toward her stomach, instead of downstream! In most cases, the contrast will barely make its way out of the colon. Jessica's intestine shot it upward.

Now we knew that the surgeons had made a very simple error: the bowel segment had been sewed in reverse. We quickly scheduled a new surgery, during which we cut through both ends of the segment, flipped it around, and reattached it in the correct configuration, confident that the full intestine would now propel food in the right direction.

I was paged from the NICU when Jessica finally pooped green for the first time. I rushed upstairs, and her parents were holding the poop in the tiny diaper as if it were a sacred object.

"I am going to bronze this stool!" her mother said, hugging one of the baby's devoted nurses.

Dr. Randolph showed up, too. He told Jessica's parents he was still kicking himself for failing to realize what had happened.

At this point I wanted to duck out of the room and sneak away. Had I shown up my boss? I knew he didn't think that way, but I felt awkward standing there. I was far less experienced than any of the doctors who had been on the case.

"And this guy," Dr. Randolph said to the parents as he pointed at me. "I heard they used to call him Flash back in Boston because he moved so slowly. But he's banished that nickname forever. I'm going to call him Fresh from now on!"

My gut tightened a bit. Fresh, as in wise guy? Smart aleck?

"Fresh eyes!" he then added.

He had assigned the task to me, but what had mattered most was his insistence that I take it from the top. Others could have solved the mystery with the same marching orders. I came to the case clear of any intellectual prejudices, and that made all the difference.

I was surprised at how supportive Jessica's parents were. There was no acrimony, no resentment or accusations. Dr. Randolph had been honest with them, and they knew that the staff was devoted to their daughter. What mattered most was that she was finally healing and on the right course.

"Never trust the notes," Dr. Randolph said, looking at us one by one. "Never trust the damn notes." He shook his head as he said it, leaving me pondering what he meant.

Solving a seemingly intractable case requires questioning the original diagnosis and all the subsequent diagnoses stemming from it. You have to question your own judgments and those of everyone around you. Dr. Randolph had essentially told us to question even him.

This collaborative interrogation—a respectful distrust—was something I had seldom seen before. But on Randolph's team it was the golden rule, and parents were critical questioners, too. Rather than being seen as disparaging or arrogant, the refrain "don't trust anyone" should be a core tenet for every doctor—and every parent. Dr. Randolph wanted every set of eyes to be probing eyes, even when they were scrutinizing his own work. To have done this in my early training would have been risky. Here it felt good and fresh and right.

CHAPTER 8:
If You Can Teach

When you are young and green and working at a teaching hospital, it takes you about two weeks to adjust to what young docs come to know as "the look." Parents will give it to you when you walk into their child's room. It begins with skepticism, transitions to incredulity, and ends in a frown of disgust. What generates it? The fact that these parents know you are fresh out of school and think you are most likely not the most experienced, and certainly not the best, doctor to be treating their child.

Were I the parent of a sick child, and not a doctor who works at a teaching hospital, I would likely have offered up the same reaction upon meeting someone like me back then. I got the look fairly often in my two-year fellowship at Children's National. But the most frightening look came from a police officer toward the end of that two years. I looked younger than most of my peers. I just couldn't conjure the gravitas of a grizzled veteran, despite having adjusted my attire and even my gait.

The police officer in question was the father of a baby whose stool was, in medical lingo, indicative of a blocked intestine. His poop was rock solid, and his obvious anguish during a bowel movement was the telltale sign of a severe intestinal crisis. As I examined him in the NICU, his father stood over me in his uniform like a guard at the gates of the White House. He greeted my every push, tug, and test on his son with a look of descending confidence in my abilities.

What I knew, but what parents like him who bring a child to a teaching hospital don't know, was that I was not going to make any final decision about what to do for his son. The attending physician, or in my case that evening the ever-present Dr. Randolph, was to be apprised of any case requiring surgery. The attending physician or head surgeon would then always direct the surgery in person, and often he would perform it with his own hands.

I had a distressing hunch that this might not be an isolated intestinal issue but something far worse—cystic fibrosis (CF). I had learned by this stage that CF usually manifests itself in toddlers through clogged lungs and infections, but in infants the disease sometimes manifests solely as a blocked intestine. Surgeons don't manage the disease, but we become involved in addressing its complications. Ever since those days at Boston Children's when I felt the parents blamed me for their son's death, I had maintained an intellectual and emotional interest in CF. Every time I spotted a patient with CF or suspected it, I wanted to attack it with all my power. Certain conditions become special challenges for doctors: you see them over and over and relate to those patients with extra intensity.

I didn't dare mention my suspicion to the father, but I knew I would have to include cystic fibrosis as a possibility, if not a probability, in offering my assessment to Dr. Randolph.

The trouble was, he was off-site that evening, at a fund-raising event for the hospital. To make matters worse, he didn't carry a pager, and cellphones were not yet commonplace. Whenever Dr. Randolph went off-site, his secretary would keep the phone number of the event handy. We knew to bother him only in the event of a real emergency—and usually had a hard time tracking him down. This was one of those moments, and the intimidating father only added to my urge to speak to him immediately.

"I believe we are going to have to operate," I told the police officer, "but I need to find my boss and get his assessment of the situation."

As soon as I had spoken, I realized how poorly I had conveyed our internal procedure. The officer's face now showed a blend of panic and disdain. I had just confirmed my inexperience or ineptness—or both.

He watched me in stony silence.

"I'll be right back," I said, trying to feign coolness as I left the room. But I knew it was too late.

We called several numbers at the club and finally, through the ingenuity of his assistant, reached the maître d'.

I described Dr. Randolph as a tall, distinguished, gray-haired man, and the maître d', to my relief, said he could spot him at his seat that very instant.

"Dr. Newman!" I heard Dr. Randolph say moments later, his tone as warm and welcoming as the first day we met.

"Dr. Randolph, I have an infant here, and I've got a hunch it's CF. I think we've got to go in pretty soon," I said. "His meconium is rock solid, but his lungs look all right. We were not able to resolve the bowel blockage with enemas, and I think he needs surgery to relieve the obstruction."

"Okay, get him prepped. I'll be right over," he said.

"And Dr. Randolph," I said. "His dad's a cop. Big guy. I get the sense he wants to see you. He wants to know who is in charge."

I heard him chuckle as I hung up—he was used to this drill by now. Parents often resist young-looking surgeons, not realizing we're just the front end of a larger team and that a senior surgeon or chief of surgery would be either meticulously supervising or performing the surgery.

I notified the team, consulted with the anesthesiologist, and did one last check of the baby's vitals. Then I went to find his dad in the waiting room. The cop's wife was still in the hospital herself after a difficult labor, and she had delegated decision making to her husband.

"We are going to have to operate, sir," I said, emphasizing the "we." He seemed to have grown taller and wider in the interlude.

"Who are *we*?" he asked. "And how many of these have *we* done?"

At that instant I spotted Dr. Randolph entering the operating room area—wearing his tuxedo from the fund-raiser. If a trumpet had announced his arrival, it would have seemed perfectly normal.

He walked up to us, and as he stuck out his hand, the cop transformed from the heavyweight champion of the world to a tired, concerned father.

"This man dresses the right way to operate on my baby boy!" he said, managing a brief laugh.

Dr. Randolph laughed, too. I sighed with relief, and the cop gave me a pat on the shoulder.

The baby did fine during the surgery, but we confirmed the diagnosis of cystic fibrosis. When he recovered, we matched him with a great team of pulmonary and CF specialists. He would require long-term care to manage his lung and intestinal issues, but new treatments were starting to make the disease manageable.

I took from the situation a lesson that I should give up trying to look older or at least wiser. I would have to live with it until I earned parents' trust. I had the inevitable chat with Dr. Randolph after the procedure. He shared with me that he had lived through similar skepticism when he was young and told me he had long battled parents' fears about teaching hospitals by being everywhere at once.

A pediatric teaching hospital is a medical center where residents and students come to learn how to care for children. All the specialties are included: ophthalmologists, oncologists, anesthesiologists, orthopedists, physical therapists, nutritionists, cardiologists, nurses, and pharmacists all get their pediatric training here. It is a hub of innovation, discovery, and inquiry based on a common commitment to advancing and improving the care of kids. The fear that green and hotshot residents will operate and care for patients with only minimal supervision plagues many of the best academic hospitals to this day. But knowing what I do, I would always want my child to be treated in a teaching hospital.

These are places where questions are constantly being asked, hypotheses tested, and debate and innovation encouraged. Pediatric teaching hospitals can seem messy and chaotic—a stream of doctors and nurses in training endlessly stopping by to poke and prod a child—but in my experience doctors discover and produce better outcomes when they are teaching and when every medical interaction is relentlessly reconsidered. Doctors working at teaching hospitals have to stay on top of every development in their field. In many instances they pioneer new forms of surgery or treatment long before they become the norm. And the success rates for procedures tend to be much higher.

Dr. Randolph used to say that being challenged by hungry upstarts made him a better doctor. He wasn't just teaching us, he was improving his own skills and judgment. Having to explain things, in the face of sharp questions and a steady stream of doubt, forces you to challenge your hypotheses and often learn something in the process.

Some years later I bumped into that police officer in Georgetown, a historic neighborhood in Washington. I spotted him across the street, keeping the raucous crowd in line on Super Bowl Sunday after the Redskins' victory. I'd had a beer or two already, so I easily summoned the courage to approach him and inquire about the health of his son.

He recognized me instantly, gave me a bear hug, and said he was holding his own despite such a tough disease. He was getting what basically amounted to a tune-up every year to clean out his lungs and reduce the risk of infection.

Then he turned serious. "You know," he said, "I would have appreciated it if you had shown up in a tux, too. It's what my little guy deserves."

He didn't laugh as he said it, and for a moment that sense of intimidation I had felt all those years before washed back over me. But then he belly-laughed and gave me another bear hug, just about squeezing the beer I had consumed right back out of me.

"Next time—hopefully there won't be one—but if there is, I promise you I'll honor him appropriately."

I've see the cop again a number of times over the years—not at the hospital but in different parts of Washington when he was out on his beat. And every time he'd bring up the tux. One time we did discuss the mechanics and benefits of teaching hospitals, and it was clear he had become a true believer.

"I didn't midjudge you, doc," he said by way of an apology of sorts. "I just judged you out of context."

CHAPTER 9:

You Never Can Tell How Far a Frog Can Jump

Pediatric teaching hospitals tend to draw superstars in niche or difficult procedures. Young doctors who want to master a certain type of cancer treatment or learn about a rare form of brain surgery will tend to identify and latch on to older masters. This is how innovation occurs: the young upstarts usually learn the skill or technique and then advance it. Dr. Randolph had developed a national reputation for several procedures, his esophageal work foremost among them. Because of that fame, we saw a lot of esophageal surgeries, and in time I felt I was developing a mastery of this procedure, too. He often had to operate on the same child multiple times, even as adults. Adjustments and complications are the norm for children who have undergone significant reconstructions, and I was at first amazed at how deep into life he tracked some of his patients.

After a couple of years at Children's National, I came to appreciate that the hospital's name didn't accurately cover the age span of the patients we were treating. Adults with conditions that had developed at birth or in childhood were not uncommon, sometimes because of the very success of the childhood treatment. Previously, patients with cystic fibrosis rarely survived childhood, but with the increasing success of treatments, they were now returning to Children's for care well into their forties and fifties. Babies born with congenital heart disease used to die in days or weeks, but now as adults in their thirties and forties, they were passing through our halls to see their lifelong cardiologists—the only ones fully capable of understanding their histories and struggles.

One of these regular returnees was a sixteen-year-old girl named Ann, whom Dr. Randolph had been operating on since she was an infant. She'd had a good run in her early teens but had undergone several interventions prior to that, the last of which resulted in Randolph's decision to abandon the flawed esophagus she had been born with and perform a total colon interposition. We would have to cut out a piece of the colon and use it as a replacement tube to bypass the esophagus. The remaining colon would be sewed back together, and the esophagus replaced. The procedure went well, but Ann returned several times after that with cases of pneumonia. Her team of doctors couldn't figure out the link, if any, between the operation and the illness. A series of imaging tests had confirmed that the reconstructed esophagus was intact and functioning properly, so the mystery deepened when she was hospitalized for pneumonia for about the sixth time in a year.

Dr. Randolph asked me once again to bring a fresh set of eyes to her case. I spent hours studying her records and radiology results. After about my tenth review of the images, I thought I saw something fishy—a shadow in the middle part of her chest cavity. I ordered another CT scan and determined from that image that a segment of her original esophagus had been left inside her. I suspected that this remnant had been filling up with mucus that was spilling over into her lungs, causing the pneumonia.

I took the images to Dr. Randolph, relayed my suspicion, and watched him as he studied the CT scan. It wasn't long before I detected a grin, which I could tell he was trying to repress. He turned to me, and I expected to hear the sort of praise that would carry me down the hall for days.

Instead, he offered up a baffling southern quip. "Well, I guess even a blind hog can root out an acorn every now and then," he said.

I grappled with the image in my head for a few seconds and couldn't come up with an appropriate retort. I had never seen a blind hog, and being compared to one brought my high to an abrupt end.

I had already seen enough doctors in my short medical lifetime to realize how many bought into the hype about having the power to fix and heal. Getting caught up in that false power, in the ego trip of saving lives and playing God, was tricky, because the gratitude of parents can be overwhelming. Being called a blind hog tended to cut short any detour into ego land.

If a personal quality could be institutionalized, Dr. Randolph was hell-bent on making humility the defining characteristic of surgeons at Children's National. But his even stricter insistence that every doctor own every case provided the real lesson in humility for me. That sense of ownership is what a parent should look for in a pediatric caregiver, be it a surgeon, a NICU nurse, or a urologist. Dr. Randolph saw it as an antidote to the increasingly impersonal, team-based medicine that was slowly starting to take over. If you were standing in front of a child, her case was yours, and you had better master every detail as if you were the first to examine her.

Another one of Dr. Randolph's favorite sayings was "You never can tell by lookin' at 'em how far a frog can jump." He would often say it when we were discussing a particularly complicated treatment or technique on a child whose future seemed in doubt. He would say it to remind us to operate with optimism, to remember we could harness the strength and natural recuperative powers of children and transform a seemingly weak frog into a champion jumper. The senior docs who practice at teaching hospitals tend to like to teach moral lessons as much as technical ones. Many of them could have left for bigger paychecks at other hospitals, but the satisfaction of teaching kept them on board. I often tell parents they shouldn't discount this dimension of pediatric teaching hospitals. The child is really getting two for one, the old master and the young upstart collaborating.

One of the most gratifying moments of my life was scrubbing for surgery with Dr. Randolph. Scrubbing is a necessary activity for infection prevention, but it also served as a sort of warm-up in Randolph's view of surgery as a team ritual. He urged us to regard ourselves as players on the field, stretching before the game, getting our heads and hearts ready for the performance ahead. I often rehearsed our surgeries with him while we scrubbed, envisioning the procedure and foreseeing the challenges.

One day while scrubbing, I decided to ask Dr. Randolph about the origins of the frog story. I had just been visiting a patient of ours who was making the kind of recovery that they make movies about. Born with innumerable problems and in Dr. Randolph's care for years, he was now a teenager in the throes of his first crush on a girl. I smiled and thought: *You never can tell how far a frog can jump.*

I had assumed Dr. Randolph had grown up hearing these animal-based aphorisms in Tennessee. As we scrubbed, I told him the story of this boy who sounded like a classic frog—he had defied the odds and was now jumping high and far—and asked where the frog aphorism had come from.

"Old Mr. Wilson would be proud of that boy," he said.

Confused, I asked who old Mr. Wilson was.

"Back when I was in med school, I was working nights at a nursing home to help pay the bills," Randolph said. "This one fella, one of the grumpiest old guys I ever met, gave me a heck of a time all year. I'd help him out of his bed, and he'd tell me I didn't have what it takes to be a doctor. I'd bring him his medicines, explain which pill was which, and he'd tell me he'd never trust me as a doctor. I'd explain a few tricks to help him manage his arthritis, and he'd tell me I didn't know what I was talking about. The day I was leaving for my residency at Harvard, I told him where I was headed, and he frowned at me and looked like he was going to spit on the ground. He was sitting in a rocking chair out in front of the residence. He looked off into the distance, and said, 'Well, I guess you never can tell from lookin' at him how far a frog can jump.'"

Dr. Randolph saw himself as a frog, too! He was, for me and many others, not so much a person as an ideal. He embodied an approach to pediatric medicine that we aspired to emulate. His ideas were frequently unorthodox and unconventional. They were about how to best serve all those kids with whom he identified as a sort of co-conspirator.

The frogs were jumping all over the place around us at Children's, and he loved it as much as a hot summer night in Nashville. It's what kept him there, and many of us who do our fellowships at children's hospitals catch the same fever. Pediatric specialists earn good livings, but the bigger bucks are elsewhere—in adult medicine and at adult-oriented hospitals. Parents should be aware of this devotion and should seek it out. Rarely in professional life today do you encounter someone accepting less pay for increased satisfaction. The enchantment of the leaping frogs accounts for this, and parents should embrace the added energy and attention that this ethos brings to the care of their kids.

Dr. Randolph was a uniquely effective motivator, but he was also a good disciplinarian when he needed to be. His reprimands still stand out for me as the most effective lessons I've ever learned, more formative in some respects than the many essential things he taught with humor.

An unforgettable one came soon after my proud discovery of Ann's esophageal remnant. A boy under our care, the son of a Baptist minister, had a complex congenital kidney malformation. The procedure to reconstruct his kidney was so tricky that the urology team, who were the primary surgeons, had called in Dr. Randolph to assist. Pediatric general surgeons like us (whose specialty is the abdomen and thorax) would get this call when other organs—in this case the intestine or the stomach—might need to be accessed to patch the kidney or construct a new bladder. What's more, Dr. Randolph had been trained both in pediatric general surgery and pediatric urology. Part of the intervention included inserting a tube in the boy's kidney and securing it to prevent an infection or reflux of urine. Even though we wouldn't usually be performing urological surgery, he asked us, his younger doctors, to witness this ourselves. He believed that a pediatric general surgeon should have a comprehensive view of surgery and care and wanted us to be prepared for all eventualities.

The day after the surgery I was doing the rounds, and I checked in on the boy. His father was there, and he seemed satisfied. The family was from North Carolina, so I started talking with them about ACC basketball.

"Y'all have got some good docs up here," he said.

I nodded proudly and said that Dr. Randolph had really seen it all, and you couldn't hope for a better mentor.

I enjoyed my chat so much that I gave only a cursory look at the boy. His vitals were fine, the incision was clean, urine was draining into the tube, and his pain was under control.

His dad and I shook hands, and I drove home soon after, pleased with the sort of people my job was allowing me to meet.

At near midnight that night, I got a call from Dr. Randolph. "Kurt, the preacher's boy," he said.

My heart dropped. What could be wrong? Did I misread a vital?

"His tube popped out," he said. "Get your fanny back in there ASAP. His father said you were the last guy who saw him!"

How Dr. Randolph could tell what I was thinking through the silence on the phone I will never understand. But I was thinking this: *I didn't insert the tube, the urologists did; my follow-up was more of a courtesy than a professional obligation. Why the hell do I have to go in at midnight when the guy who did the procedure is sitting at home watching a basketball game?*

"You own the case, Kurt," Dr. Randolph said before I could think of something to say.

During my twenty-minute return drive, I kept trying to understand his logic. Didn't the urologists own the case—and the mistake? Wouldn't the lesson of accountability be better spent on them?

By the time I finished reinserting the tube, it must have been around two a.m. I walked back into the waiting room and saw the boy's father there, wide awake. And suddenly, feeling that father's immeasurable love for his boy, I understood what Dr. Randolph wanted me to understand: whatever we touch, we are entirely accountable for.

I had not exercised the appropriate care in my examination. That meant I owned the tube failure just as much as the guys who had inserted it ineffectively in the first place. I had not removed the dressing to check the stitches and ensure that the tube was effectively secured. Randolph's reprimand stuck with me, as it did with almost everyone who worked with him. The Randolph ethic—a homespun blend of humility, optimism, and diligence—was built on total accountability.

His words—"You own it, Kurt"—would ring in my ears for the rest of my career. The compulsion to own it, to improve the life of any child he came into contact with, whether as primary surgeon or consulting physician, was what set Dr. Randolph apart. I've learned to look for that compulsion and accountability in my own children's caregivers, in new hires, and in my staff and assistants. It didn't come naturally to me, but I came to appreciate that it is the founding premise of superior pediatric care.

On another occasion I returned home late one night and, going through my mail, noticed a letter in Dr. Randolph's handwriting. I opened it, hoping for a congratulatory note of some sort from my mentor.

I poured myself a beer in my tiny kitchen—it must have been ten o'clock at night—and, eager to take that first sip after a hard day, took the index card from the envelope.

I flipped it over, and taped to it were eight stitches—precisely eight—and knew right away what I had done this time.

I had recently performed neck surgery on a young boy to remove a cyst, and I had closed the incision with eight stitches. Those eight stitches were to stay in for no more than five days, as stitches on the face and neck that remain longer tend to cause visible scarring—the sort of "railroad tracks" that can become a point of teasing and shame for children once they become self-conscious and encounter the cruel world of school. There is so much blood flow in the neck, face, and head that it requires fewer than the usual seven or eight days to heal.

I had forgotten to instruct the boy's parents to return to the clinic on the fifth day to remove the stitches. I never did figure out how Dr. Randolph discovered my mistake, or how he came to be the one to remove the stitches, and I was too embarrassed to ask. But I had run afoul of one of the norms he taught us in caring for children—a dedication to preventing scarring. Just as he insisted that a psychiatrist be included on any case that might impact a child's self-esteem, Randolph was ever mindful of the way a child will develop both physically and emotionally. He didn't want a patient, five or ten or twenty or fifty years out, to see the physical scar, but he was also thinking about mental scars and urged us to ensure that whatever happened in the hospital didn't affect a child's healthy development down the road.

Not long after Dr. Randolph's wordless rebuke, I saw a seven-year-old girl with brain cancer. My job was to surgically insert a special IV into a major vein in her chest, through which her chemotherapy chemicals would pass. When we finished her exam, I sat with her mother and pinpointed the spot where I would insert the IV. The spot was relatively high and to the left of her chest.

I turned to her mother and smiled. "That way when she wears her first prom dress, no one will see the scar. We'll do our very best to minimize the scarring, too."

Then I turned to the girl. For the first time, I tugged down my collar a bit and showed her the scar from my own thyroid cancer surgery back when I was in medical school.

"Yours is going to look a lot better than this, but I just wanted you to see I've got one, too." I said. "It's not so bad, really."

The girl studied my scar, I winked at her, and she smiled for the first time.

I said the line matter-of-factly, letting it drop with Randolphian understatement.

I would never contemplate scar tissue with carelessness again. And once my young patients grew up and started sending me prom and wedding pictures, I would realize how right my teacher was.

CHAPTER 10:
How to Hold a Baby

One measure of how far pediatric surgery has come over the course of my career has nothing to do with children and everything to do with medical tradition. Dr. Kathryn Anderson was a senior surgeon at Children's National when I arrived, and it was immediately obvious that she was the most technically proficient surgeon on the staff. She was British, and her crisp accent was all the more effective on a surgical staff that included a couple of twanging southerners.

What I did not know for most of those first two years was that Dr. Anderson had broken pediatric surgery's glass ceiling. In 1964, when she finished near the top of her class at Harvard Medical School, she had been told point-blank by one of the chiefs of surgery at Harvard that there would never be a slot for a female in the surgical department there. She spent a year as a pediatric resident at Boston Children's, but her husband, a pioneering medical researcher, had accepted a position at the National Institutes of Health, so they moved to Washington. She was selected for a full residency in adult general surgery at Georgetown University Hospital. Following that, she wanted to train in pediatric surgery, so she applied for the fellowship program at Children's National while working at Georgetown.

Now I hope I haven't made Dr. Randolph look saintly, though I realize

I've made him look darn good. He had some flaws, most of which were the product of his intensity or, as in this case, of attitudes that were common to his generation. He told Dr. Anderson what the chiefs of surgery at Harvard had told her: there was no room for a woman in the OR, and certainly not in their training programs.

I cringe when I think about this now, knowing the impressive contributions so many female surgeons have made to our hospital. But Dr. Randolph quickly got his comeuppance. Late in the summer, he was left with an empty slot in his program when a candidate suddenly changed his career plan. By this point he had already formulated his surgical schedule and staff. A gap of one meant a breakdown in the entire structure.

I would give anything to have been in his office as he rehearsed his phone call to Dr. Anderson. He told me later that he had been able to sense her keen talent the first time they'd spoken about how to perform certain procedures, and deep down he had been kicking himself for not hiring her then. Legend has it that Dr. Anderson took his call, discussed the issue with courtesy, then made him cool his heels for a couple of days awaiting her answer. She coveted the gig, but she had decided to teach him a lesson.

A few months into my fellowship, she had taught me a lesson, too—one of the most enduring ones of my formative years as a surgeon. I was sitting with a group of surgeons in the cafeteria one afternoon after a morning in the OR, and we were discussing the intricacies of a bowel operation we had just performed on a newborn. I thought of a similar case I had worked on at the Brigham, and I waited for a pause in the story swapping to bring it up.

"Well, back in Boston we . . ."

Ka-boom.

Dr. Anderson laughed sharply. "Please don't say 'back in Boston,'" she said. "I assure you I have nothing against the place, but I'd prefer you focus on learning what we are going to teach you here."

I wondered what she meant.

"You don't know babies yet," she said. "You know adults and you know kids pretty well, but you don't know babies. And for the sake of the babies here, please don't pretend that you do."

I can still feel how the blood rushed to my face. I'd had six months of pediatric surgery experience, even less neonatal experience, and up to that point I had operated on very few babies.

My colleagues tried to change the subject. We all knew that Dr. Anderson was not only a great pediatric surgeon but one of the best neonatal surgeons in the nation. It was more than her dexterity, I realized. There was something insanely communicative in the way she touched and held newborns. Dr. Randolph's gregariousness and goodwill were most effective with older kids, but Dr. Anderson was the Zen master with babies. The more I watched her operate and compared her technique and success rates with those of other surgeons operating on infants, the more I began to think that in an ideal world there would be hospitals exclusively devoted not just to pediatrics but to neonatal medicine.

Babies are that different from children, as different biologically and anatomically as children are from adults. Medical intervention on infants, from surgical strategy to the calibration of anesthesia, from pain measurement to pain control, is completely different. Newborns' organs are immature and developing rapidly. We still have so little knowledge about the impact of our interventions on them. We are discovering only now that the brain of a newborn is in such a state of flux at birth that the chemicals used in anesthesia may impact its natural development. Neonatal neuroscience is forcing us to reassess all early-life interventions and how we perform them.

Babies obviously exhibit a positive response to cuddling and touch, and there is an emerging effort to incorporate these techniques into the recovery protocol. We used to insist on the same sterile environment maintained in adult medicine in the NICU, ignoring the newborn's craving for physical connection. But recent research has proven we were wrong. Twenty years ago in NICUs, babies were completely confined to their isolettes; today we encourage nurses and parents to hold them at scheduled intervals. Dr. Anderson understood these biological and psychological differences and needs long before they were generally recognized, and she adjusted her surgical technique, prescriptive care, and even her touch and voice to take them into account.

It was commonplace for me to go up to the NICU to see a patient and spot Dr. Anderson there, holding a baby and gently rocking her. The way she examined babies was unique, too. She used an extraordinarily precise touch to probe for a mass or organ. She studied not only a baby's face but his or her entire body for signs of pain. When she operated on a newborn, her incisions and the way she moved tissue were gentle and deliberate. The nurses were the first to recognize Dr. Anderson's particular skill with infants. I noticed that they would often discreetly call her for a consultation, even if she wasn't the baby's doctor.

Dr. Anderson was the surgical leader of the team that introduced ECMO (extracorporeal membrane oxygenation) to Children's National. Along with Dr. Billie Short, the head of the NICU, she had successfully performed the first surgery at Children's National using ECMO in 1984. The technology is used for babies who are not able to breathe on their own or exchange oxygen. The ECMO machine takes blood from a vein, sends it through its own artificial lung, suffuses the blood with oxygen, and then returns that oxygenated blood through a tube connected to the artery.

The original ECMO machine looked like a contraption from a 1950s science fiction film, or a low budget version of *Star Wars.* A tangle of tubes, cylinders, pumps, water heaters, and monitors hanging on a couple of steel poles, it made the sort of funny noises you'd expect from the invention of a mad scientist when you plugged it in and the thing started chugging and pumping. In the 1970s Dr. Robert Bartlett realized that, with a couple tweaks, the machine could serve young babies with lung problems. The idea was to relieve their lungs of the duty to perform for a few days and allow the lungs to develop more fully without the stress of having to supply a new life with oxygen. While the heart develops early, as any parent who has seen a sonogram knows, the lungs are usually the final organs to fully mature.

Babies' lungs are filled with liquid while they are in the womb—a fetus gets its oxygen supply from the placenta. At birth, and only at birth, the lungs kick in as the child ejects all fluid and instantly starts to use its spanking new little oxygen pumps. That's why that first wail after a baby is born is always a good sign.

Getting the ECMO pump in place called for tricky surgery to connect the machine's plastic tubing, or cannula, with the carotid artery and the jugular vein. Dr. Anderson performed the operation in the NICU rather than the operating room to avoid transporting very sick babies.

It wasn't long before I was asked to assist her on an ECMO procedure. I was paged just as I was carrying my dinner tray in the cafeteria. I left the tray, full, on a table and rushed up to the NICU, still an alien place for me, despite my efforts to learn from Dr. Anderson's reprimand. I had read the ECMO manuals and had rehearsed the procedure in the lab, but this was only the second baby to be placed on ECMO in the history of the hospital, and everyone felt the pressure. As I was scrubbing and awaiting Dr. Anderson's arrival, I experienced a level of anxiety I had never felt before, not even on my first surgery.

Dr. Anderson had made it clear that she would be the surgeon for all ECMO cases until the team had been adequately trained and the outcomes were consistently perfect. This meant that she would be the attending on probably the first thirty or so cases. I knew she would be in the driver's seat this time, but I didn't want to let her down.

That night, because we were in the NICU, the light was bugging me: it was not as clear and bright as in the OR. My positioning and stance felt awkward, too, as the nurses and technologists jostled around me to get the pump ready. There was an urgency in the air, and I grew even more anxious.

As I waited for Dr. Anderson to arrive from home, I felt sweat dripping down my torso and back. The NICU was kept at a higher temperature than the rest of the hospital, to accommodate babies' need for warmth. The headlight around my head felt too tight and was giving me a headache. The whole situation felt off and unsettling. I worried that this did not bode well for the procedure. The NICU, which was on the third floor of the hospital, had wide windows overlooking the surrounding neighborhood. I glanced out the windows and spotted a pool complex where swimmers were frolicking as the sun set. I longed to dive in with them.

Dr. Anderson at this point walked calmly into the room in her scrubs. She assessed everyone's position, checked the machine, and studied the baby closely.

"Okay, Kurt, please prep her neck," she said in her crisp English accent.

When you are a surgeon, you can quickly assess the technical ability of another surgeon. From the first time I operated with her, it was evident to me that Dr. Anderson was a consummate technical surgeon. She made no wasted move. Hers was a complete economy of motion. She could anticipate her colleagues' moves, too. I quickly caught her rhythm as she made her first incision.

We promptly identified the carotid artery and the jugular vein and assessed their caliber. Dr. Anderson chose the tubes to be inserted into the blood vessels. There was no room for one bad move. A slight error could result in a damaged blood vessel, making hookup to the machine impossible. A momentary lapse could introduce air bubbles into the ECMO circuit and trigger a stroke. Dr. Anderson had the benefit of delicate hands and fine fingers, so she could access tight spots that most surgeons struggled with. She also set the surgical field up perfectly—the drapes, the height of the table, and the positioning of the patient fit like a tight puzzle.

As we moved through the operation, time stopped, and the art of the procedure took over. Dr. Anderson's calm focus relaxed me, and I quickly forgot about my anxiety and self-doubt. After about fifteen minutes, she paused for a second and nodded.

"Go ahead and complete the hookup to the heart-lung bypass machine," she told me.

I did so and watched the baby's skin color turn from dark blue to pink. We stood in place as the technicians took a quick X-ray to verify the correct placement of the tubes while Dr. Anderson studied the baby's motions and responses.

Dr. Anderson would go on to become surgeon in chief at Children's

Hospital Los Angeles, one of America's best pediatric centers. Later she became the first female president of the American College of Surgeons. Her legacy at our hospital was the prioritization of neonatal surgery and care. Neonatal surgery is its own niche within pediatric surgery, as thousands of parents in the United States discover every year when their babies are born with complications. Specialized neonatal medicine provides one of the most decisive arguments for pediatric hospitals. Dr. Anderson's instruction still guides me today as a CEO as we work to create the NICU of the future, determined to harness new technology while emphasizing intimacy and care.

CHAPTER 11:

"There Are No Conflicts of Interest Here"

One morning when I had been at Children's National for two years as a fellow, Dr. Randolph called me into his office. Usually this happened when fellows were ending their training and the time had come to discuss their future job placement and career. I had a slight hope that I would be offered a permanent position, but the staff was full at the time, and I had steeled myself for disappointment and another job search.

"Kurt, I'd like you to consider becoming a permanent part of our surgical staff," Dr. Randolph said, without so much as asking how my day was going. "How would you feel about that?"

I couldn't figure out if he was so courteous that he felt obliged to ask a question to which he surely knew the answer, or if he was simply incapable of presumption. Was he actually *asking* me if I wanted to become a part of his team? It was absurd. They already had a full complement of surgeons, and I had nowhere near the skill or experience of his three partners.

"Well, I know I'm supposed to say, 'Let me think about it,'" I said. He stared at me, unblinking. "But Dr. Randolph, I accept."

I expected a hug or at least a hearty handshake. But he acted as if I had given him a blood pressure reading.

"The thing is," he said at last, "now you've got to realize you aren't just a surgeon anymore. You're in charge. You own every detail now. It's a whole 'nother league, Kurt."

I thought back to the first interview, when Dr. Randolph had revealed his early struggles instead of hitting me with zinger questions. No meeting with this guy ever turned out the way you expected. He was surgeon in chief, in charge of all the surgeons, operating rooms, anesthesiologists, and OR budgets. But I was no longer his assistant, and he was making that quite clear. *Attending* in medical parlance means that you are tending to the patient as your own, but it also entails taking responsibility for teaching fellows. That was the most startling thing for me as I walked out of his office: I would now be charged with teaching new trainees, just as Dr. Randolph had taught me. I found that to be much more of a challenge than taking full responsibility for managing my own cases. But there would be one last case where I would need Dr. Randolph.

A year or so into my new life as an attending physician, a call awakened me at two a.m. After a dozen years of disrupted doctor sleep, my nervous system had learned not to leap at the sound of the phone. Before that cold winter night, if you'd asked me whether I felt confident in my abilities as a surgeon, I would've answered, a bit cockily, yes. I'd been in surgical training for over eight years. I had been the chief resident at Brigham and Women's Hospital in Boston and had taken care of hundreds of very sick patients. During my nearly two years as a fellow at Children's National, I'd fixed ruptured blood vessels, repaired livers damaged by bullets, removed tumors from kids' kidneys, cut open the chests of newborns, and grafted skin onto children with burns all over their bodies.

And yet a doctor can never be fully equipped mentally and emotionally. Surgery, even in today's hypermodern OR, still holds surprises. The human body never ceases to offer up new mysteries and challenges.

"Dr. Newman, we have a three-day-old newborn who's losing heart and lung function rapidly," the nurse said on the other end of the line. "The neonatologist is with the boy now. She believes we have to get the child on ECMO before the night is through."

"I'll be right over," I said.

I'll be right over. Doctors learn that line pretty quickly. It's part promise and part dodge, true but sufficiently vague. It's one of the few lines from medicine that the movies get right. We doctors say it regularly to nurses, other doctors, trauma technicians, and even desperate parents. We say it patiently, confidently, and sometimes deceptively. We say it, more than anything, impulsively and because we know we have to.

I read Tom Wolfe's *The Right Stuff* when it came out in 1979. I liked the book, not least because it so accurately captured that leap certain professionals have to make in high-risk situations. You get all the training in the world, you perform the task a thousand times in simulation, with an expert watching over your shoulder, but when it comes time to go to the moon, you realize you haven't done it before. Only a few guys have ever gone to the moon. And only a few surgeons have ever cut open a friend's newborn infant. Astronauts risk their own lives, but surgeons risk someone else's life—in my field, the life of someone's child.

That night as I made my way down Georgia Avenue in the darkness through the blinking red lights, I caught myself driving way too fast. I recognized the *Right Stuff* adrenaline rush, the same thing Chuck Yeager and John Glenn craved, and told myself to knock it off. It would surely do me no good in surgery. Then I reprimanded myself again. I'd already committed an error: I'd forgotten to ask the boy's name. I never wanted to become a mere technician, and I loathed the way surgery sometimes encourages that sort of dehumanization. I'd made a habit of asking the child's name on every emergency call, and as I raced into the special parking space for on-call surgeons, I was beating myself up pretty good. *Have you ever seen Randolph not have a child's name on the tip of his tongue?* I thought angrily.

I hurried into the hospital, found the nurse waiting for me, and resisted the impulse to switch to autopilot. I paused, and because everyone was ready to go and I'd finally arrived after what felt like hours, that pause felt eternal.

"What is the baby's name?" I asked.

The nurse seemed startled for a second, then looked down at the chart. "Evan McNamara."

The name sounded familiar. I repeated it a few times in my head as I headed toward the NICU operating room. At this point adrenaline kicked in again, and I quickly rehearsed the ECMO installment in my head. The actual operation isn't the most challenging part. You expose the carotid artery and jugular vein in a baby's neck, insert catheters into them so blood will be drained from the heart and stripped of carbon dioxide, and then ECMO fills the blood with oxygen and pumps it back through the artery. You rely on the skilled team around you to make sure the blood is the right temperature, thin enough, free of air bubbles, and pumping at the right pace. What's challenging is that the baby is usually very sick, losing pulmonary and possibly cardiac function. You're not in a pure OR environment, as this procedure is usually performed in the NICU without the lighting and amenities of a true operating room. You hope no impure air or infection sneaks into the child through the surgery or the machine.

I'd been the surgeon on multiple ECMOs by now and still marveled at that shining moment when the dark, almost black, blood that's been drained from the baby in one catheter goes back in bright red. For a moment, you're witnessing the miracle of life itself.

When critical surgery is at hand, a doctor will feel as if he's shooting straight down a high-speed assembly line with the child on a well-lit table at the end. The surgeon rushes through the doors to the OR, and nurses have his scrubs and cap waiting. A doctor, usually a fellow or resident on shift that night, walks beside him to the sink and briefs him on what he has seen and knows thus far. Another nurse has the correct size of glove hanging from her own gloved hands as he turns and slips his hands into them. The anesthesiologist starts talking the minute the surgeon enters the prep room. Human interaction is reduced to the sparsest, most precise conversation imaginable.

But that night, once I had prepped, I took a shortcut through the NICU via a little waiting area adjacent to it. I suppose I thought there'd be no one there at three a.m. I knew the boy's name now; I knew what had to be done. But to my shock, as I crossed the waiting room, I saw a good friend of mine, Bob McNamara.

Suddenly it all came back to me. A few weeks earlier I'd gone to the Kennedy Center in downtown Washington to see one of my favorite singers, George Jones. (I love country music.) It was a wonderful show, and as I was walking out, humming, I slowed down as a pregnant woman turned in front of me to cut across the hallway. I heard her say my name. I looked up and recognized Bob's wife, Carol, surely in her third trimester.

I'd known Carol since our college days at the University of North Carolina. She was one of those people whom everyone knew and loved to be around because she was always so upbeat. More than once during gloomy days in Boston I'd recall her walking across The Pit outside the student union or passing by on Franklin Street, her sunny optimism radiating. We ran in the same circles in Washington, and she always took an interest in my work. That night after the concert, as the crowd pushed us along, she'd quickly updated me on her pregnancy, and I wished her and Bob well.

Now here was Bob pacing in the NICU waiting room. I hadn't yet quite registered that I was about to cut into his newborn son's neck.

"What are you doing here?" I said, before my brain processed the obvious.

"I think you're about to operate on my son," Bob said sheepishly, ending his sentence just as I mentally finished it for him.

I did the only thing I could. I grasped his shoulder and tried to summon the most confident face I could. I nodded, patted him on the back, and walked into the OR. We surgeons do this backslapping and the like because language so often fails in such situations. What do you say, especially when you're a science guy who read Shakespeare as a freshman in college but since then has been nose-deep in anatomy tomes?

Now it was up to me to save their baby. Neither med school nor my training had prepared me to operate on the child of a friend.

I reprepped and strode up to Evan, that little life lying there in the spotlight. Every time I approach the operating table, I feel as if I'm stepping up to some sort of altar. It's an honor and a privilege to have parents entrust you with the life of their child. It's also an overwhelming responsibility, and that last glimpse of worry on Bob's face passed through my head as I made the first cut into his son.

Evan's lungs needed a break, a respite from the stress of delivering oxygen to his imperiled body. We weren't sure what the problem was, but by placing him on ECMO, we could give his lungs a chance to develop as we tried to get to the root of the problem.

We finished the operation, and Evan seemed to be stable. ECMO requires a nurse or technician to monitor it constantly for air bubbles. If a stray air bubble were to pass from the machine into Evan's artery, it could go right to his brain and kill him. So we set Evan up at a station in the NICU and prepared for the usual waiting and watching. Our hope was that his lungs would respond within days, exchanging oxygen and carbon dioxide on their own and slowly assuming control of breathing away from the machine. We could measure this by slowly decreasing the amount of support provided by the machine and putting more responsibility on the lungs. The real test would be to temporarily turn the machine off to see if the heart and lungs could sustain breathing on their own.

But they didn't. It was clear after a couple of minutes that Evan's lungs weren't kicking in enough to keep up with his oxygen requirements.

While the procedure did seem to increase his oxygen supply and stabilize him slightly, we didn't see the improvement in overall oxygen measurements and distribution that we were hoping for. Even with the support of ECMO, for some reason he wasn't able to process and supply the necessary oxygen to his organs.

It eventually became clear, after a battery of tests, that Evan had a profound and likely intractable metabolic problem. He probably had an undetectable genetic flaw that impeded the chemical processes upon which life depends. We suspected there was an issue with his liver's ability to break down iron. Elevated iron levels pointed directly to liver trouble, and we had to do a biopsy on his baby liver—a very stressful test for a newborn's system—to figure out if we were right. Our far-fetched hope was that the biopsy would tell us he had a condition that was correctable.

The liver is an organ that regenerates, so normally taking a snip of liver for a biopsy, or even a big chunk in case of cancer, isn't too much of a problem. The nature of the organ gives you some leeway. You try to take as little as possible, but you do so with the confidence that the organ will take care of itself. That's the good news.

The bad news is that a young child's organs are so fundamentally different in their development, functioning, responsiveness, and even texture from an adult's that infants may as well be considered a human subspecies. That reality, insufficiently understood, accounts for the existence of pediatric surgery as its own unique discipline.

For babies of Evan's age, performing a biopsy on a liver is like cutting several clean lines into a small glob of jelly, taking a slice out, and then stitching the jelly back together. Any one of these three steps runs the risk of causing irreparable bleeding; all three taken together pose one of the most daunting challenges in pediatric surgery. Jelly is, by its essence, virtually unstitchable.

Our only option, while not wholly impossible, was certainly a dismal last resort. I walked the halls of the hospital after our team had settled on the procedure. Normally, this sort of walk energizes me. Just as an old football player loves the gridiron or a fisherman loves the wharf or a horse trainer loves the stables, I love the hurly-burly of hospital life, the snippets of passing conversation, the collegiality, even the antiseptic smell and the fluorescent light.

But that day I felt as if I were walking in a foreign country. All sounds were distant and muffled. No face came into focus.

How could I perform such a high-risk procedure on the child of a friend? By this point, I'd spoken with Carol and Bob countless times during the week. They were conducting themselves with a grace that I found both wholly inspiring and entirely unfathomable. I had their total support. And yet imagining myself having to leave the OR and tell them Evan hadn't survived shook me to my core.

One impulse overcame me: I had to call Dr. Randolph. Even though I was relying on him less as I grew, Evan's situation—or more precisely, my situation—called for his intervention. One of the many benefits of a pediatric specialty center is that its institutional memory, and hopefully its mentoring system as well, make black swans—those rare crises that, on an annual basis, are not so rare when you look at total numbers and not percentages—a little less menacing.

Our team had agreed to wait twenty-four hours so that Evan could stabilize prior to the surgery. I was off duty that day, and in the evening I drove out to Dulles Airport, an hour west of Washington, to pick up a friend. My anxiety about the upcoming procedure was so severe that I had a bad headache. I gripped the steering wheel too hard and felt my hands sweating. Finally I pulled over and picked up my heavy early-model car phone and called Dr. Randolph.

I stumbled over his name when he answered. Once I'd become an attending surgeon, he'd told me I should start calling him Jud. The transition from formality to friendship was a hard one, and when I could summon the single syllable, Jud, I usually croaked it out. Mostly I'd just stopped using any form of address, but this time I reverted to deference mode.

"Dr. Randolph, I can't do this McNamara surgery," I said, somehow confident that he knew what I was talking about and would recognize my voice. Just getting the words out was a relief.

The connection was full of static, and his voice was choppy. I couldn't understand his first response, so I rambled on about the complexity and risks involved in the surgery, which of course he already knew. I named other surgeons who would surely be up to the task and would probably perform better than I could, which I really didn't believe for a second. And I continued to circle around my discomfort at the idea of operating on the child of friends, of people I knew personally and would have to face over and over again after the surgery, even if, God forbid, something went wrong. Dr. Randolph began to respond once or twice, but the static overrode him, so I just kept babbling nervously and, for the most part I'm sure, incoherently.

"I think it's unethical, frankly," I said as I wrapped up my speech, somehow convinced that'd I'd come off as logical. "My relationship with them excludes me. We're just too close. I don't think I ought to be the one to do this."

Suddenly the connection improved, and Dr. Randolph's voice sharpened. His southern drawl and slow, steady speech came through loud and clear.

"Dr. Newman," he said, "there is no surgeon in this world who will do a better job on that baby than you. And that is because you care about him and the family so much. There are no conflicts of interest here. Now get back there and do it."

And with that he hung up. Cars were whirring by, and my own car shook when trucks passed. I was shaking slightly, too. Dr. Randolph hadn't even hesitated, and I felt a rush of energy and confidence.

I picked up the phone again to call a cab for my friend, whom I'd just left stranded at Dulles. Then I made one last call, to the OR, to tell them to prep Evan for surgery right away. He had stabilized, and there would be no difference between tonight and tomorrow morning. I turned the car around and, making a concerted effort to stay within the speed limit, drove back to Children's.

On my way to the scrub room, I detoured to the waiting room, intentionally this time. I knew Evan's parents would be there, and I wanted to talk with them—more for myself, I think, than for them. I wanted to feel their support and peace one more time prior to the operation.

I was not aware of their religious sensibility or allegiances, and I was not particularly prone to prayer. But spontaneously, in the cold and empty waiting room in the stillness of the nighttime hospital, we held hands and prayed silently. We looked each other in the eyes, and their simple nods were the only real blessing I needed.

I walked into the OR and saw Evan on the table with the anesthesiologist, who was beginning her administration. This alone is a challenging task in a child of this age. For starters, a baby's veins are so small that often you can't see them to set up the intravenous administration. The calculation of an effective drug dosage is more challenging due to a baby's weight in any instance—let alone a sick baby who's lost weight or been born prematurely. Selecting the type and size of the breathing tube is tricky. Determining the moment to begin surgery is more complicated than in an adult, too. Are the muscles paralyzed? Are the pupils reactive? Do the vital signs show that the anesthesia has taken hold? And then, once all this has been determined, the balancing of medication throughout the procedure begins. One step too far, and a baby, far more quickly than an adult, can stop breathing.

As I cut into Evan's abdomen, a nurse prepared a special gelatin sponge, a sort of Styrofoam substance that we apply to the cut edge of the liver. We then drip through pipettes a gel that hardens slightly as a buttress against a raw, bleeding liver. All around the sponge's edges we sprinkle a powder that promotes clotting. Then once the tiny area has hardened, we can try to apply sutures.

Evan's liver was visible now, so tiny and wobbly, like a jellyfish or a glob of yogurt. Athletes speak of being in the zone, and that's where I found myself. Whatever that state was, it helped my team and me pull off the biopsy. The stitching, one of the most challenging surgical procedures I'd done in my young career, took hold. Bleeding was minimal, then it stopped altogether. The procedure had gone as well as could be hoped, and we agreed we could stitch Evan's abdomen back up.

Having avoided the catastrophe I'd been so anxious about, I strode out into the waiting area and made an entirely different error. I felt I'd just beaten some incredible set of odds. Elated at the success of the procedure, I allowed Evan's parents, my friends, to rejoice. Tears of joy flowed from their eyes, and they hugged each other and me. But this is where I did them a disservice. I'd failed to sufficiently emphasize that this was merely the successful *first step* in a process that could bring them the worst news: that Evan's metabolic system could not support his body and organs, that Evan could not live without life support. I should have tried to minimize their joy, but I didn't have the heart to do it. I had seen and felt their suffering, and I didn't want to steal this respite from them.

Several days later we learned that the biopsy had demonstrated clearly that Evan's metabolic system could not process iron. One of the fundamental nutrients needed by the human body, iron can also overwhelm the body, especially one as young and precarious as Evan's. The liver, which in the body is equivalent to the water treatment plants we see on the outskirts of cities and towns, breaks down iron. But Evan's liver couldn't do that. The waste, or in this case the excess, couldn't be processed, so it kept floating around Evan's system and would eventually crowd out all other nutrients.

Oddly, the finality of the biopsy made my next meeting with my friends easier. Biology had rendered its final verdict, and there had to be some consolation for them in that.

As we sat in a tiny room adjacent to the NICU, I tried to explain in the voice of a friend and not a surgeon what the neonatologist had already told them: the flaw in their son's metabolism and the impossibility of improving it. Bob and Carol made it easy. I'd never seen, nor thought conceivable, such grace in the face of anguish.

"We just don't have enough, we don't have enough," I said. I still don't know entirely what I meant. They were just words, not empty but not going anywhere either.

"Thank you so much for being there for our son," Carol said.

And then, for the first time in my career, a child's parents asked me to pray over their infant's tiny body with them before we ended life support.

We went to Evan's room. We circled around his quiet incubator. The heat warmed my forearms and chest. His parents held hands, and each took one of mine. No one said anything. They closed their eyes first, and I followed. Our silence together was the prayer.

A few days later, knowing I was still hurting, Dr. Randolph stopped me in the hall.

"That family has peace, Kurt, knowing that you, their friend, did everything you could," he said. "If they can face life without their son, if they can get to that point, your being part of it will help them immensely. It will help them heal."

I have operated on more than fifty children of friends since then, and I've lost a couple more. Each time Dr. Randolph's assurance that no one can treat a friend's child better than a friend has empowered me. Despite the loss, I felt better for having owned the case. Some of the most rewarding moments of my career have come when working with friends in an effort to deliver their children to better health.

PART II:

Vital Lessons

CHAPTER 12:
Old School

I was coming of age as a surgeon just as technology and insurance companies were eroding the old-fashioned one-on-one relationship between a pediatrician and a child and his or her family. It was getting harder—not just for us hospital folk but for the doctors on the front lines—to fulfill Dr. Randolph's injunction to own each and every case. Pediatric practices, increasingly structured as business partnerships managed by accountants rather than doctors, started to use electronic records as an excuse to eliminate the pediatrician-child partnership in favor of efficiency. Children could now see any pediatrician in a practice, and the net result was that they no longer had their own exclusive doctor following them through their fevers and accidents, keeping track of their behavioral and psychological development, and watching them grow.

Dr. Beale Ong was a soft-spoken pediatrician who referred many of his patients to Children's National during my early years on staff. He was thoroughly up to date in his knowledge and treatment plans, but he was defiantly old school in his hands-on approach to interacting with his patients and with us at the hospital. He would prove to me that, even in an age of email and electronic files, the bridge between hospital and pediatricians can be critical to success.

But I was not always so admiring of him.

My Boston days had instilled in me a mild chauvinism about surgery. I had interacted primarily with surgeons, both professionally and socially, and had lived in a world where surgeons' names were on buildings, wings, floors, rooms, and books. It was impossible to be entirely inured. Even after many years in Washington, I secretly believed in our superiority, but I would soon learn just how mistaken I was.

Dr. Randolph, as you might imagine, beat most of that attitude out of me pretty quickly. More than his harangues, his relationship with Dr. Ong showed me the folly of my ways. Whenever Dr. Randolph was around Dr. Ong, his demeanor changed. He was deferential, spoke more quietly—and generally seemed happier and more at ease. You could feel the respect they had for each other. They taught me how a hospital and frontline pediatric practices could function in lockstep.

Quick to smile but slow to wisecrack, Dr. Ong rarely engaged in small talk. He had well-combed silvery hair, wore better suits than any surgeon, and interacted with everyone with even more graciousness than Dr. Randolph. Like most good doctors, he realized that the successful practice of medicine depends not just on assessing a patient's immediate symptoms but on factoring in their full medical and life story. He was a master questioner, probing the child and his or her parents until he developed a picture not just of the case but of the patient.

Long before the field of hospitalist medicine (a hospitalist is a staff physician in charge of managing a patient's care in the hospital) emerged, Dr. Ong seemed almost to be a full-time member of the hospital staff. But he wasn't—he was very much in private practice, following generations of kids and their families. I had often heard him consult on cases but had never worked with him directly until one day I received a call from one of the surgical secretaries saying that Dr. Ong needed to speak with me urgently.

Truth be told, I was a little annoyed. I was making rounds and had to complete them before heading into surgery for the afternoon. The slightest disruption would make me rush a patient visit.

I spotted a phone outside one of my patients' rooms and decided to call Dr. Ong, to keep Dr. Randolph happy. I was already reflecting the bias of the coming wave of med school grads, who would find regular interaction with referring physicians foreign or just plain irritating.

"How are you, Dr. Newman?" Dr. Ong asked courteously.

"Fine," I said curtly.

"I just sent a young girl over to you who does have a history of stomachaches," he continued, as polite as ever, "but this time I think it really is an appy. I've run her through our protocol here and would appreciate your insight."

Today, so long as the frontline doctor catches it in time, we can usually do an ultrasound or CT scan and diagnose appendicitis without surgery, thanks to the accuracy of imaging. Many physicians now wait and monitor the progress of the appendicitis (or an appy) before rushing in to operate. Emerging protocols are even investigating a strategy of using antibiotics exclusively and not operating at all. But back in the 1980s and early 1990s, surgeons lived by the 10 percent rule: you performed surgery, and you'd better be wrong at least 10 percent of the time to be safe. Wrong, in this case, meant not finding appendicitis—so you'd performed an operation to confirm that you didn't need to operate. The reason to operate was to prevent a ruptured appendix down the road. Surgery was the only way to ensure the safety of the child, for a ruptured appendix was (and still is) life threatening.

When I found the girl and her mother, I was sufficiently uncertain about the diagnosis to want to wait and see if the symptoms presented themselves more clearly. In other words, I didn't trust Dr. Ong.

I told the girl's mother this was my plan.

"Wait a minute," she said abruptly. "You wouldn't want to miss an appendicitis and have it rupture on my daughter, would you, Dr. Newman?"

Dr. Ong had told her about the 10 percent rule and had coached her on what to ask me and what support to give for her case.

I was a little taken aback, but her knowledgeable intervention pushed me to reconsider. "I sure wouldn't," I said.

I looked at the girl's tummy again, weighed the odds, and said, "Young lady, we're going to operate."

The girl nodded with a small smile. I had never before had a child nod at the mention of surgery, but she had clearly been prepared for what was to come. Dr. Ong had made the right call: she did have appendicitis, and we caught it in time.

I called him as soon as I finished the procedure.

"That mother sure knew her medicine, didn't she?" he said with a slight air of mischief in his voice.

Playing along, I said, "I wonder if she went to the Ong school of medicine."

A pediatrician's intimate knowledge of the strategies and personnel of a hospital can be fundamental—even lifesaving. The more I witnessed the benefits that came from a seamless collaboration between hospital and pediatrician, the more I came to rue the fact that technology, cost management, and insurance companies were militating against it. Dr. Ong had taught me to seek out and listen to pediatricians, but the kind of relationship he had with us is something that was becoming harder and harder to find.

A few years later I examined a boy whom Dr. Ong also felt might have appendicitis, and even though only a few of the checklist symptoms were evident, I called him to suggest that we operate. I assumed he would ask me if I had consulted with Dr. Randolph, so prior to the call, I had done so. As I informed Dr. Ong of my hunch and presented my argument for operating, he said something that still rings in my ears:

"How wonderful it is when we are all on the same page—you guys there at the hospital and those of us out here on the front lines!"

The practice Dr. Ong shared with Dr. Frank Stroud was renowned as one the best pediatric practices in town, and it had served multiple generations of families. Sometimes today, as medicine has grown more decentralized and specialized and as collaboration among doctors is rarer and more difficult, I marvel at our level of coordination and trust.

At the heart of the relationship was a common view of our roles as guardians of the children of our community. I once told Dr. Randolph that I was stunned by the extent to which he consulted with Dr. Ong and Dr. Stroud.

He looked at me impatiently. “We owe it to the kid, Newman,” he said sharply. “He’s got a long life in front of him. Dr. Ong wants to make his practice a multigenerational business.”

Good pediatricians realize how slippery the symptoms of many conditions can be. In some instances, the symptoms are steadily apparent, but sometimes they come and go. That can be frustrating for parents—and challenging for the frontline pediatrician trying to nail down a diagnosis.

Diagnosing a hernia in a baby or child is one such tricky case. The cardinal symptom is intermittent swelling in the groin area. The swelling may be there when the pediatrician examines the child—but it may not be. Such hernias, more common in boys than in girls, can become life threatening if the abdominal organs get caught and twisted in the hernia.

I used to love those cases because the operation is so satisfying. I enjoyed talking through the problem with parents, showing them where the hernia was, and explaining how it could be fixed. I would show them how the muscles did not seal off, allowing a small hole to form, through which the intestines could poke through. I would describe how, during surgery, we would find that opening and close it off with a few stitches so that the hernia would not come back. I would always describe the possible complications—in boys the risk of injury to the microscopic vas deferens, which lies nearby, and in girls possible injury to the ovary. I promised them I would take care of their child—even to the point of describing how the stitches would be placed underneath the skin to ensure minimal scarring. It was so satisfying to reassure a scared family about what the surgery on their child was going to be like.

But to reach that point, careful choreography with a pediatrician we could trust was fundamental. The swelling was rarely present when the child came to the surgery office for examination. I had to rely on the history provided by the parent or the pediatrician.

This is where the trust would come in. If a pediatrician like Dr. Ong, who paid fastidious attention to his patients, told me he had seen swelling, I could take him at his word and act as if I had seen it myself. If he had not seen the hernia, then I would generally insist upon seeing it myself. This could mean evaluating the child for a month or two.

And it worked both ways. As an attending surgeon, I kept my beeper on all the time and told the office staff that if a pediatrician called, I wanted to take that call myself. I wanted every pediatrician to know that I was available to talk things over. I also wanted them to keep me from screwing up. Pediatricians like Dr. Ong had so much critical information about each child that might have seemed ancillary but was really essential. What allergies might a child have? What psychological issues? What clues should I be looking for in their reactions, speech, and gestures?

Dr. Randolph's earlier lesson—that I had to own every case I touched—had been driven home by Dr. Ong. And based on my experiences with Dr. Ong and other pediatricians who embraced the same code, when parents asked what they should look for in a pediatrician, I began advising them. The way Dr. Ong practiced pediatrics was becoming almost impossible given the paradox of medicine today. The centralization of electronic records and insurance billing and the establishing of medical networks has actually caused a decentralization of pediatric care. Today it is harder to find that one person who knows a child's health history inside out. Dr. Ong would find it difficult to get through to a child's hospital team, and surely he would struggle to find the time to visit his hospitalized patients.

But ironically, old school is also cutting-edge today, and I know several pediatricians who manage to stay engaged with the team involved in a hospitalized child's case. More and more children's hospitals are serving as catalysts to fully integrate primary care into their continuum of care. So I advise parents to seek out pediatric practices that serve as a medical home, where pediatric specialists and a children's hospital are part of the medical neighborhood. Parents considering a pediatrician should ask several key questions: Where would you advise we take our child in case of hospitalization, and what are your relationships there? Can I call you if my child is hospitalized? Can I put you in touch with my child's surgeon or specialist? Is anyone in your practice available in the middle of the night in case of an emergency?

CHAPTER 13:
Maternal Instinct

In the spring of 1989 I fell in love with a NICU nurse at Children's National named Alison. She happened to have attended Vanderbilt University, so she passed muster with Dr. Randolph, a Nashville native and graduate of Vanderbilt and its medical school.

One night Alison and I were at a wedding reception for a friend when halfway through the first toast, I received a page. I quietly excused myself, found a pay phone, and called in. The operator told me an infant had been born with severe intestinal issues several hours earlier at another hospital. Tyler, she told me, needed emergency surgery. I rushed back to the reception and suggested to Alison that she come with me. I told her I'd drive her back to her apartment in northern Virginia afterward. I wanted both to impress her with my skill and to prolong our date.

When we arrived, I got into my scrubs while the surgical fellow briefed me on the issues Tyler was facing. Alison checked in with the nurses and donned sterile garb, too. We walked into the OR together, and I began my routine: I checked to see that the team was in place, double-checked the instruments, took a final look at the X-rays and vitals, and for a moment took in the child in front of me. Then I proceeded with my first cut.

Tyler had been born with his intestines and abdominal organs splayed outward. They had formed outside his abdominal wall so that they sat exposed on top of his midsection with no skin protecting them. There was also some duplication: he had a double appendix and two intestines. I had never seen anything like it—not only was such a thing not in the textbooks, I had never even heard it described when my colleagues swapped stories in the surgeons' lounge.

I took a step back and decided to call Dr. Randolph, not as a mentee but as a desperate attending surgeon. I had somewhat successfully learned to interact with him as our surgeon in chief, and like the other four attending surgeons on staff, I still sought out my old teacher for advice. I described the situation and waited to hear what he would say.

He paused and cleared his throat.

I pushed the phone into my ear.

"Well, Kurt, I guess on this one, you're on your own," he said.

He didn't laugh. Nor did I. And I still don't know if he was testing me or confident that I was up to the challenge.

With extreme cases like Tyler's, the immediate surgical objective is to build mechanisms for the removal of stool and urine, then to stabilize the baby for future surgical reconstructions. The key, as usual, was to do no harm. Here that meant removing as little of the intestine as possible. Our initial goal was to get Tyler through the first few days of his life. It was a long shot, but we had to try.

I had called one of our top pediatric urologists, Dr. Gil Rushton, to assist in the case. When he arrived, we methodically turned Tyler's intestines and bladder inward and stitched them into whole, albeit crude, organs. We inserted a catheter for the urine and created an ileostomy to collect his digestive waste in an external bag. When we closed him up, we were fully aware that he would face a battery of surgeries in coming years just to keep on living. I hadn't looked at Alison once during the operation, but I was confident I had impressed her with my coolness and savvy. I was much less confident that Tyler would live more than a few months.

As Alison and I walked back to the car. I slowly came out of my surgical haze and waited for her to marvel either at the scale of the boy's problems or,

I hoped, at the methodical ingenuity with which we'd addressed them. Instead, I got walloped. She told me she couldn't fathom what she'd seen when we walked into the OR.

I didn't know what she meant. What she must have seen was standard: an infant alone on the operating table under blazing lights while the anesthesiologist prepared his equipment, the nurses prepared their spaces, and I read the records one last time.

"Can't you see that you guys left the baby alone when he most needed solace?" she asked in a challenging tone. "Who was monitoring his body temperature before you administered anesthesia? Didn't you realize how cold that room was? Who was talking to him, cooing to him? I wanted to hold him while you were all so busy with your routine."

She was right, of course. The temperature of operating rooms is borderline frigid, but I'd never given it, or the aloneness of the child, a thought. As we drove, she kept at it. In my mind's eye, I saw the ending I had envisioned to our date—an admiring glance, maybe even a kiss—slipping away. I stayed silent, trying to think of a way to change the subject.

"And who are you," she continued, "to think a baby doesn't need company under such stress? They're way more emotionally intelligent than you surgeons realize! I can guarantee you that boy was experiencing unimaginable stress. Just because he couldn't tell you about it doesn't mean it wasn't happening."

The night didn't end well, but the overall story does. I married Alison in 1992 and never again left a baby or child so alone prior to surgery. Dr. Randolph attended our wedding and was the life of the party, but he retired that year at sixty-five. A surgeon, like an airline pilot, is expected to go gracefully at that age, for the need for reflexes and stamina conspire to make surgery a relatively young person's game. He missed Tennessee and had always planned to "not stick around past my welcome," as I heard him say a few times. He had decided to teach part time at Meharry Medical College in Nashville, where he could mentor minority medical students interested in pediatric medicine and surgery.

I was pleased for him, but I spent his final few months at Children's in denial and disbelief. I had developed my skills and mind-set under him and hadn't fully conceived of life at the hospital without him. Losing him meant, I supposed, having to grow up once and for all. But more than anything, I lamented the massive loss for the children of our community. He said I was on my own, but I felt he was leaving the kids on their own, too, and I didn't think any combination of attending surgeons, including me, could plug the hole.

Alison's reprimand was unsettling but also motivating. Now that we have had two children together, I believe it wasn't just the NICU nurse but the future mother in her that grew so alarmed that night. In the past couple of decades, medicine has taken significant leaps when it comes to diagnosing children's health issues and coming up with a comprehensive and humane plan for remediation. But in our race to reinvent our field, in my opinion, we've thrown not the baby but the *mother* out with the bathwater.

For me, the mother's opinion, typically unscientific but thoroughly rooted in a powerful capacity for intuition and empathy, became a key tool in assessing, calibrating, and treating a child's disease or trauma. I realize that in these politically correct times I should include the father in the equation, and I have seen some fathers with incredible intuition. But the insight, hunches, and sixth sense of the person who has given birth to a child often stand out as remarkable contributions to a medical plan. This doesn't mean mothers are always right. Often parents will come to us with an emphatic idea of what is wrong, and one of the first things you learn as a doctor—even before the wave of Internet-based home diagnoses—is to be skeptical of the first report. You can't jump to conclusions too early, and you need to question every note and recollection. But a parent's story, and most frequently a mother's, can often provide details, observations, intuitions, and even suggestions that prove fundamental to success.

I was reminded of this lesson a few years later, when a family walked into my office and I was struck by the intense gaze of the older of the two women.

She stared at me, unblinking, while her pregnant daughter sat across from me and told me her story. Their respective husbands had taken the chairs behind them. The daughter, in her fourth month of pregnancy, had been told by her obstetrician that a cyst had been found on the fetus's lung and that terminating the pregnancy was her only option. They'd come to me to find out if any experimental surgical option existed.

As she talked, I could sense that she harbored doubts about the medical advice she had received. She didn't trust in her gut the recommended course. And as she talked, I sensed her mother watching over her. The grandmother-to-be had a ferocity about her, a primal protectiveness that dominated the room.

When the daughter finished, the older woman leaned slightly forward. It was her turn to speak. "We have come here not for a second opinion but for an expert opinion," she said.

That was it. One sentence, and I heard my marching orders loud and clear. The mother's carriage and manner were refined, her posture ramrod straight, her clothing and jewelry formal and precise. Her leadership role in this family was obvious. We doctors can be intimidated by the most unsuspecting candidates, and that was the case here. I realized I was essentially dealing with two mothers, a confused young mother-to-be and a wise, experienced veteran who trusted her daughter's instincts.

I asked for the ultrasound scans, which the young woman had been holding tightly in her hands. I told the family I would go downstairs to study them with one of our top radiologists. No one said a word or moved as I left the exam room.

Second opinions are precarious for doctors, and this was the first time I'd been asked for one involving a recommendation to terminate a pregnancy. As I walked downstairs to the radiology department, I couldn't shake the image of that commanding matriarch. Something about her determination rattled me. Despite my absolute commitment to objective professionalism, she'd succeeded in compelling me to scrutinize the scans with a predisposition to her point of view.

We've had a number of great radiologists at Children's, but that day I was especially pleased that Dr. Dorothy Bulas was on duty. A skilled radiologist, I'd learned long before, is part forensic detective and part art critic. On a tour of Washington's National Gallery of Art one day with a docent, the analogy came to me clearly. The way the docent described paintings and captured their textures and nuances transported me instantly to the radiology room. On television and in movies, we see an X-ray go up, and the doctor opines quickly, as if you could get so good at this stuff that it comes lickety-split, with no room for indecision. The reality is not so snappy. The trick, I learned from watching professionals like Dr. Bulas, is to let the answers come to you as if you were studying a great painting.

Dr. Bulas took the images, placed them on the light box, and considered what she saw before her. I'd learned to track her eyes with mine. I could follow her focus, direct mine to the same point, and somehow pick up on the workings of her brain, just a foot from mine. You could almost hear the debate in her head as she measured the tumor, determined its proximity and threat to the heart, and tried to project its course of growth.

The tumor was distant enough from the heart and seemed to be in its own plane of tissue. She measured the size and volume with a caliper built into the scan.

She kept looking silently, formulating her opinion.

"No need to terminate," she said, with no more gravitas than if she'd told me what kind of dressing she wanted on her salad. I was stunned, as much by her statement as by her confidence. "The ratio of lung to tumor size will surely increase in the final two months of fetal development. The pregnancy should be fine, but you may have to operate after birth."

In essence, the cyst, formally known as a congenital cystic adenomatoid malformation, would likely remain static in size and severity. It was what it was going to be. We had a strong track record with treating these sorts of cysts successfully and knew this type tended to grow little, even in the final weeks of fetal development, as babies pack on pounds. As the baby's lungs continued to grow, the size of the cyst relative to the size of the lungs would decrease. This, she reasoned, would allow for a decent degree of lung functioning at birth. The rest we could fix in due time.

I went back upstairs to share the news with the family. As I walked into the room, I got a sense that no one had spoken since I'd left the room. The grandmother sat in precisely the same position as when I'd left.

"We believe the odds of a positive outcome are greater than a negative one here," I said cautiously to the expectant mother. "Your baby shouldn't have any problems immediately, though soon after birth we'll likely want to consider surgery to remove the cyst."

As I spoke, I realized that what I was saying would be confounding. We were confident; the obstetrician had been confident: someone had to be wrong, either us or the obstetrician. The stakes were obviously high.

The grandmother-to-be nodded matter-of-factly as her daughter turned to embrace her husband. Then she smiled, suddenly sweet and warm. Her daughter's hunch had spurred her defiance, and they had both saved a life.

During most interactions, we doctors run several scenarios simultaneously in our brains, and as we discussed next steps and said goodbye, I was already preparing myself for the call that would come next.

A few days later, as expected, I spoke with the upset obstetrician. She'd just met with the family and told them they were making a big mistake. She told me I was doing them a disservice.

When I hung up, I grabbed the ultrasounds they'd left with me, walked back down to the radiology room, and clipped the sheet to the light box. I sat looking at the images, with a vision of that matriarch flashing before me. Had these women swayed me too much? Had I pressured our radiologist? Had that family's desire to proceed with the pregnancy overridden my better judgment?

A couple of months later I got a call from the mother-to-be. Her baby was scheduled to be delivered by a cesarean section, and the family and the obstetrician requested that I be there in case emergency surgery was necessary. I had consulting privileges at the delivery hospital, so her request was both feasible and intelligent.

That day I drove across town, marveling at the good fortune of this infant. Her mother had defied the medical establishment. Her intuition had bested conventional wisdom. This was a pattern I would witness again and again throughout my career. It isn't always mothers—it can be fathers, sisters, aunts, and grandparents. Dr. Randolph's point was to expand your team of "informants" and advisers as widely and intelligently as possible. But mothers are typically the most intuitive.

The delivery went fine. The baby was stable and did not need emergency surgery.

Over the years I ran into the family matriarch several times. "How did you know," I asked her once, "that your grandchild was going to make it?"

She smiled, amused, and said simply, "Maternal instinct once removed."

Her lesson stuck with me. Over the rest of my surgical career, I would try to do something they never tell you to do in medical school: aggressively incorporate a child's family, and particularly the mother, into my team. In pediatric surgery the stakes are so high and the lives in some instances so new that there really is only one expert on that young life in the room.

In twenty-five years as a pediatric surgeon, I've rarely encountered a mother who will take the first bad news as the final decision. But most do know when it's time to let go. A mother is suited, even programmed, to monitor that fine line between justifiable risk and excessive intervention. It is rare to encounter a mother who does not know when to stop a treatment or forgo an operation. Likewise, most will also recognize when we have done all we can do and it is time to stop.

A woman who conceives a child, carries and delivers a child, and then begins to nurture that child has lived through the most physiologically and spiritually powerful event a human being can experience. Her instincts with regard to her offspring are acute, and it behooves doctors and nurses to assess her capability as a team member and seek out her opinions. Sometimes in medicine we so aspire to be cutting-edge that we lose focus of obvious and natural assets right in front of our noses.

CHAPTER 14:
Trauma

Children's National is only about a three-mile drive from the White House, but we work in an alternative universe. A futuristic structure of glass and steel, the hospital sits on a high plane to the north of the great dome of the Capitol. The McMillan Reservoir down below feels like a moat between the bustle of city life and the hospital. But the city has an unfortunate way of keeping us connected with events taking place in its streets. The accidents and injuries that our emergency department treats every hour of every day are a stark reminder both of the risky lives of children and of the uniqueness of their needs and responses.

Trauma is the leading killer of children. Each year in the United States, according to Safe Kids Worldwide, an organization linked to our hospital, preventable injuries kill eight thousand children, and nine million children are treated in emergency departments. The lesson: as a parent you are likely to end up, sooner or later, in the emergency room. An emergency room that exclusively sees children is more adept at pediatric trauma care. From the type and size of medical equipment to the skills acquired by doctors and nurses through repetition, the ER is another clear case of the need for children's specialty centers.

In the last year of my surgery residency in Boston, I had received a call from Dr. Marty Eichelberger, the head of trauma surgery at Children's

National. I was well aware of his growing reputation in the field and had briefly met him during my interview. We exchanged a few pleasantries, and I wondered why he'd called.

"This is not a quiz. I just wanted to ask if you know what the leading killer of kids is," he said at last.

I paused, mentally ran through a list of the diseases I had come across at Boston Children's, and realized my time to answer had passed.

"Trauma," he said bluntly.

The answer seemed obvious, but I had never thought of accidents as a disease. In fact, the word he used to describe pediatric emergency room visits and trauma surgery was *pandemic.* He went on to cite the statistics, ran me through the calamities of his previous day to make the data more concrete, and urged me to spend a good part of my time and energy in the coming months getting ready for emergency pediatric surgery.

I had done a few trauma rotations at the Brigham, and I'd regularly volunteered in the ER when I was a student at Duke, so I'd had my fair share of car crashes and shootings. But the numbers were startling. Dr. Eichelberger spoke about statistical probability, not possibility, and I thought of all the stunned parents I had encountered in my brief experience in the ER.

Children's trauma is its own realm of medicine, with distinct nuances and complications. In most hospitals with trauma centers, the emergency department doesn't distinguish between children and adults. Teens with broken arms sit alongside alcoholics with damaged livers in the waiting room; mothers cradle babies with pneumonia in their arms as paramedics rush a sixty-something heart attack victim past them on a stretcher. At the Children's National trauma center, it is all kids all the time, and I found this both logical and intimidating. That many kids suffered from emergencies? I was shocked.

Keeping this conversation with Dr. Eichelberger in the back of my head, I tried to work my way into trauma cases whenever I could. As I paid closer attention, I came to appreciate that every dimension of trauma surgery is different for kids, from the assessment and treatment of shock to the patterns of injury to the healing capacity of organs. What it took to treat and save an endangered young life was nothing like what it took for an adult.

During my first major trauma case at Children's National, Dr. Eichelberger's call came back to me. A three-year-old boy had been in a car crash with his family, in a child seat. He came in with the emergency crew, and as we began the protocol, his vital signs looked stable. Members of the trauma team began the assessment process. A cool professionalism descended over the room as the nurses took the vital signs and called them out. It looked as though the child had had some head trauma—he had a bruise on his forehead—but I was confident that I had everything under control.

But I broke the first rule of trauma care: check that the airway is intact. As the lead surgeon in the room, this was my job. For any initial assessment, the mantra is airway, breathing, circulation (ABC). This is as true for adults as it is for children. I had assumed from the boy's healthy color and stable vital signs that there were no airway issues, but an emergency room pediatrician on the trauma team who was listening to his chest suddenly said she couldn't hear any breathing sounds on the left side.

"Come on," I said brusquely, "how can that be? He looks good and there's no sign of a problem with his airway."

"Take another look!" the pediatrician snapped.

I opened the boy's mouth and saw that he was missing a few teeth. I looked around inside and saw some blood but no teeth.

The pediatrician and I stared at each other for a second. "He aspirated his teeth!" she hissed impatiently.

I took a laryngoscope and probed the back of the child's mouth, examining his throat and vocal cords and the opening of the trachea. There were a couple of teeth there, which I grasped gingerly with forceps. I then suctioned out the blood, which improved his breathing. The child "pinked up" with the return of oxygen. The missing teeth had been preventing him from breathing.

I felt sick to my stomach, appalled at my failure to heed the first cardinal rule of an emergency room physician.

We rapidly placed an endotracheal tube so that we could have a secure airway, and everything else checked out fine; we performed a CT scan of the head, and the image showed no bleeding or injury. But we also ordered a chest X-ray, and sure enough, we found another tooth down in his left main stem bronchus. We would have to retrieve the tooth to prevent an infection or lung damage. This was not a simple procedure—the airway of a child is narrow, and the tooth was slippery.

At this point I remembered Dr. Eichelberger's telephone call. Trauma, I realized, could take many forms—insidious, sneaky, and seemingly minor at first. As often as not, it isn't worthy of a TV drama. You always have to be on the lookout for unexpected signs—especially in children.

I learned that day that a child can appear deceptively normal in the aftermath of an injury. That lesson served me well over the years. I would soon encounter toddlers with severe respiratory distress whose parents had not even realized they'd swiped some peanuts from the counter or ingested an earring.

One night not long after the case of the missing teeth, I was on call and received word that a girl had a blocked airway and likely needed surgery. I raced to the hospital, took my usual shortcut through the waiting room outside the operating room, and spotted a familiar face—an old high school friend. I was thrilled to see her, forgetting for a second our location and its implications.

"But what are you doing here?" I finally asked.

"My child inhaled a peanut, and they just told me they might have to operate!" She began to tremble, then caught herself. "What are you doing here?"

"Well, I'm a pediatric surgeon," I said. "It looks like your daughter may be my patient—I'll be right back."

We spent over an hour trying to pull that peanut out. In fact, we weren't even certain afterward that we had removed all of it, since the girl still complained of breathing difficulty. We went back a day later to make sure it was completely removed—and found a tiny piece of peanut lodged in the right lower lobe bronchus, the portion of the airway that is the conduit for air to the right lung.

Airway emergencies are some of the most challenging cases for pediatric surgeons. For me, it was always one of the trickiest tasks to maintain the right level of anesthesia while using a scope to fish out a peanut, a toy, or a button. Since the anesthesia is administered through the same airway the surgeon is working on, the surgeon can breathe in leakage of the anesthetizing gas. I've gotten some nasty headaches this way and have occasionally been halfway anesthetized, so the relief of holding that absurd piece of flotsam up is always palpable. A child's survival can hinge on which trauma center the ambulance brings her to.

The day began with one of those clear, cool, blue-sky mornings that put an extra bounce in your step. I was subbing on trauma duty for the surgical fellow, who had a brief appointment outside the hospital. The trauma team was highly practiced and disciplined, consisting of the attending surgeon, a fellow, a few residents, nurses, an anesthesiologist, and a radiologist. I was in the NICU making rounds when my beeper went off. The neonatal nurses, protective of their tiny patients with extreme sensitivity to noise, leveled unappreciative stares my way. I tensed up.

The trauma center was looking for me. A fourteen-year-old girl had been shot in the chest in the nearby neighborhood of Capitol Hill. She had had a pulse when the EMTs put her in the ambulance, but they could no longer detect it and she had stopped breathing. As the EMTs rushed her to the hospital, they were performing CPR to attempt to resuscitate her.

The best-case scenario, I reckoned, was that the patient was in shock from blood having seeped into the pericardium, the membrane around the heart. The pericardium is a tough membrane. It contains about twenty milliliters of the clear, serumlike fluid in which the heart is suspended. It's as if the heart were in a womb that lubricates it and keeps it from banging against the lungs and ribs. This fluid-filled sac, which usually protects the heart, oppresses it in a condition called pericardial tamponade. If this wasn't the explanation for the girl's being in shock, there would probably be no way to revive her.

As I rushed downstairs to the emergency room, I rehearsed our inevitable and immediate task. Even before we administered anesthesia, before we took her vitals or assessed her condition, we'd have to cut her chest and rib cage wide open, to instantaneously relieve the pressure around her heart. In other words, the moment we saw her, we would have to start cutting. The odds were one in ten thousand that what was stopping the heart from beating was accumulated blood—not a bullet or overwhelming internal bleeding. It was our only hope.

I rehearsed the steps in my head as we waited for the girl to arrive. The resident, the nurses, and I would all be ready with the requisite surgical equipment in hand. After making a huge cut through the tissue and muscles between her ribs, we'd clamp everything back. Another doctor would then use huge shears to cut through her sternum. Then we'd insert a big retractor, and I would start turning the circle crank that protruded from it. As I did, the girl's rib cage would slowly open, tearing apart blood vessels and tissue. The assisting doctor would again use the shears to cut through the ribs and bone. Then we would place several large clamps on the jutting tissue, bones, and muscle to keep everything wide open. The whole process would take a couple of minutes.

This kind of incision is highly controversial. You do it only if you suspect (or in this case, hope for) a pericardial tamponade—a condition in which blood or fluid collects in the pericardium and exerts enough pressure to keep the heart from beating. I'd done this type of procedure a few times before, and it had never worked. Some doctors view it as too brutal, too hopeless, given the low probability of success. I bet it leads to saving a life one time out of every hundred it's attempted.

But even if the procedure is successful, it merely gives you an opportunity to restart the heart. By no means does it fix all the organs potentially damaged by the prolonged loss of blood flow. So the procedure forces us to confront our obligations as doctors: Do you go for it all, pull out all the stops to save a child's life, and disregard the larger ethical debate? Or do you concede to probability and let a life pass? Even more, do you subject a child to this sort of radical intervention? Since adults are more often the victims of gun violence, it was more common to do this procedure next door at the Washington Hospital Center, but here at a pediatric center?

We didn't ask ourselves these questions in the moment the EMTs burst through the emergency room doors. One paramedic was pumping on the girl's chest. Another was bagging her with oxygen. For a split second, I looked up at her face and then took in her body. Long and lean, she looked like a runner or a basketball player. Someone was dousing her in antiseptic fluid. I was just trying to make sure I didn't cut anyone as I lifted up my big scalpel. We easily got her chest open, and the instant the heart was revealed I could tell that the pericardium was tense.

We saw that blood had built up in the pericardium surrounding the heart, and that pressure from the bloated pericardium was preventing the heart from beating and sending blood out to the body and its organs. I knew full well that the chest compressions by the EMTs had been having no effect.

I used a scissors to open the pericardium to relieve the trapped blood. I put one hand in back of the heart and one in front and started to gently milk the organ, pushing from the bottom up to get any of its remaining blood out to the body. This is essentially the most direct version of CPR there is. You take the heart in your hand and gently squeeze it, hoping it will catch your rhythm and, when you stop, maintain a semblance of that rhythm. You're reminding the heart how to beat. I was not squeezing the life out of her but trying to squeeze life back into her.

Meanwhile, the team was pumping blood into her veins to her heart through IV bags full of O negative, the universal blood type. I looked up and saw that instead of letting the bags drain naturally, my colleagues were literally squeezing the blood out of the IVs, toothpaste style, to create enough volume in her circulatory system so the blood would reach her heart. It started to pass through, and I was tempted to squeeze her heart just as hard to pump the blood to the rest of her body. But I had to remain gentle. A nurse was now administering various medications to stimulate the heart further, hoping it would start beating on its own.

After a few seconds, the muscle felt right to me, alive somehow. I stopped massaging and saw the slightest tremor. This turned into a tiny beating that slowly picked up its pace on its own. But then as her heart slowly turned red again, arcs of blood squirted out of a tiny hole in its top left quadrant. I impulsively put my finger over the hole and squeezed again. This time her heart kept beating, but no blood shot out. I kept my finger there, directly on the barely beating heart of a fourteen-year-old gunshot victim, and realized two things right away: she was as lucky a person as there was on the planet that day, and we needed to get a heart surgeon as quickly as possible. We looked closely at her heart (the size, as in most kids her age, of the average adult male fist) and saw that the bullet had passed through the pericardium and into the right ventricle. It had missed her coronary arteries—which would have produced a major heart attack. The bullet was of a small enough caliber not to have blown the muscle tissue of the heart apart.

I stood there for about five minutes, her warm heart pulsing steadily against my gloved index finger. The surgical team stood by while we waited for the heart surgeon to rush down from the cardiac care center to help me stitch up the hole. I looked at her face again as I stood there.

Her name, I later learned, was Tanessa Starnes, and she was the double Dutch champion of her age group in the city. She was a good student, and on that pleasant May afternoon she'd been jumping rope on a school playground prior to a tutoring session.

The sport she was involved in might have saved her life. Her heart muscle was stronger than most, able to withstand the trauma. Her body was better able to tolerate oxygen deprivation and lactic acid buildup. As an athlete, she had obviously stressed her system for fun innumerable times, and that had prepared her to withstand the unimaginable stress of a bullet to the heart.

When the heart surgeon, Dr. Frank Midgley, arrived, we barely needed to speak. When surgeons with a good rapport work together, it's like two musicians in a great duet following the same sheet music. As I moved my finger slightly, he put one stitch in, then another as I moved my finger again, then a third as I moved my fingertip to the very edge of where the hole had been. I slowly removed my finger, and he placed one final stitch. We both watched as this lovely red organ pumped life throughout her body again.

But even now that we had restored her heart function, we feared that Tanessa had spent so much time without blood flow that her brain and other organs might be damaged permanently. She hadn't bled when we cut her open, and my brain did the math. She'd likely been in the ambulance for a minimum of twenty minutes, and her heart probably stopped beating halfway through the trip. Fifteen minutes is a critical marker—that is when brain damage likely starts to ensue. Had we pulled off a Hail Mary surgery, as they called odds-defying passes at the end of football games, only to now be foiled by the time it had taken to get the patient here?

The team wheeled her up to a proper operating room to clean her up, close the incision, and insert tubes into her chest to drain the blood. After that she'd go to the ICU, and the waiting game would begin. We now faced the ethical fallout of our decision to save her life. Would she have a decent life? Or had so much time without blood flow damaged her brain and other organs?

That night I drove to her Capitol Hill neighborhood—I'd lived a few blocks away in my first year in Washington. I saw a playground and imagined her skipping rope there earlier that day. The sight made me angry. Would she ever run around here again?

Until Tanessa woke up, we'd have no clue about her higher brain function. I called in during the night, and the nurse told me they could already see primitive reflexes (those emanating from her brain stem) returning: she was starting to produce urine, her heart was maintaining proper blood pressure, and she reacted to touch. But until she was awake, we wouldn't know if she could think or speak properly.

Because I wasn't yet a parent myself, I'd never felt the oppressiveness of a wait like this one. This lull, this waiting—they don't train surgeons for it. Decision, action, and then results—that's the progression we internalize, and when it is thrown off kilter, our impatience rivals in its power any other emotion.

Late the next day I went to the ICU to see her. As I turned the corner to her bed, I put my hand on her foot and looked up at her angular face. Even with the breathing tube in her mouth, she managed a huge smile that knocked my socks off. She was alone and relaxed, and yet clearly, almost palpably, alive and eager to get back to jumping rope. She didn't yet have the energy to speak, but as she smiled at me from her bed, the weight of my ethical distress and uncertainty began to lift. This girl was going to return to a fully functioning life. Her big, healthy spirit was going to bounce back quickly.

Tanessa was wide awake in thirty-six hours. She was breathing on her own in three days and was walking the halls in five. We'd rolled the dice and won, and a big part of our calculus from the very beginning had been her youth. Had she been twenty years old, she probably wouldn't have completely recovered. Had she been thirty or older, her prognosis would have been worse. The resilience of a child's body makes pediatric surgeons look better than we are. Tanessa had been dead; now she was alive. My job had been not to restore her life but simply to make the fixes that would allow her life force to reassert itself. Something about the upward ascent of biology, the cellular lust for life in young people, amazes me to this day.

I'd entered pediatric medicine with a special interest in thyroid surgery because of my own cancer in medical school, and here I was suddenly dealing with a bullet to a child's heart. I knew trauma surgery would be a part of the work at any urban hospital, but I hadn't grasped the depth of the social and socioeconomic crises that were being delivered to our door every day. And I'd never imagined the frequency with which I would be operating on children who were little more than the collateral damage of violent adult behavior.

Pediatric trauma surgery is even more demanding of specialization and repetition than general pediatric surgery. And yet at midnight at a hospital anywhere in America, when a child is severely hurt in an accident, the high probability is that those attempting to save that child's life will be a surgeon and doctors trained in adult medicine. Why can't our health care system establish a pediatric trauma system that acknowledges the direct correlation between the experienced pediatric ER providers and successful outcomes in child trauma? Why wasn't this even being talked about? The answer to Dr. Eichelberger's question about the leading cause of death among children has become obvious to me, and so has a simple way to reduce the number of trauma deaths. On October 7, 2002, I grasped better than ever the randomness of pediatric accidents and catastrophes. At the time, Washington, D.C., was being terrorized by a pair of men who were killing people at random around the region using a high-powered rifle. On that Monday morning, about twenty miles from Children's National, a young boy was dropped off by a family member at his middle school in Prince George's County, Maryland. As he got out of the car, he suddenly fell to the ground, and the sound of a rifle echoed. The sniper had hit the boy in the chest. The family member knew enough to quickly realize that he had been shot. Instead of waiting for an ambulance, she raced him to an urgent care center nearby. When she got there, a doctor immediately began resuscitating the boy and called the Maryland State Police for emergency transport. He had an IV and a chest tube inserted by the time the helicopter arrived to transport him to Children's National.

Fifteen minutes later, we could hear the helicopter landing on the helipad on our roof. Dr. Eichelberger and I, who were the attending surgeons that day, were waiting for him with our team in the operating room. We prepped him for surgery, quickly opened his chest and then his abdomen, and I remember thinking that it looked as if a bomb had gone off inside him. I worried that he had suffered too much tissue damage to survive.

Dr. Eichelberger was the lead surgeon, and he'd operated at Bethesda Naval Hospital (now the National Naval Medical Center and part of Walter Reed National Military Center) in the past.

"It looks like this boy is back from the battlefield," he said.

His lungs, diaphragm, and liver had suffered immense damage, but we were able to control the bleeding and repair the different organ injuries one by one. Once the surgery was completed, he was transferred to the intensive care unit. Within days he took full hold of life again and began to thrive. Each time I examined him I marveled, recalling my days treating adult gunshot wounds back in Boston. This boy was a stunning example of the phenomenal recuperative power of kids.

He did quite well over the coming weeks, though he had to recover in the hospital under an alias because the two terror suspects were still at large.

I saw a longtime OR nurse with a slightly older child who had attended the same school not long after he was discharged, and she just kept shaking her head in disbelief at what had happened.

"I've taken care of so many kids, but until it happens to someone you know, you never appreciate just how important a children's hospital is," she said. "There should be one in every city in America."

CHAPTER 15:
That Phantom Pain

I was bent over my desk catching a catnap, which we surgeons learn to do on a dime, when from my doorway a confident female voice asked, "How are you?"

I looked up, expecting to see a strong, no-nonsense woman in her mid-twenties and was shocked to find a child who couldn't have been older than thirteen. My assistant gave me a quick smile as the girl announced herself and walked right in. She was one of the most cinematic young patients I'd ever encountered. She had Julia Roberts's hair and Lauren Bacall's sophistication. I thought, *I hope my son ends up with someone like her.*

She wore a big red hat, a Kentucky Derby concoction that made her look not so much like a 1950s movie star as like a teenage girl trying to look like a 1950s movie star. She wore a red scarf to match and various necklaces with colored beads snaked around it. Every time she moved, the beads clanked, and she shook her arms to adjust her bracelets. This girl was commanding. Her eyes—big dark circles that seemed to fill up half her face—seemed not to blink. She kept shifting her long hair with her braceleted hands so that there was always a little jingle.

"I'm Victoria," she offered coyly.

"Nice to meet you, Victoria," I said, realizing now that she had been on my schedule. Her parents had warned us that she liked to handle her doctors' meetings herself. "How are you today?"

"I am fine," she said. "How are *you* today?"

Victoria was now cancer free after years of chemotherapy and radiation, but those treatments had left her with a phantasmagorical and seemingly incurable disease: pain. Pain inhabited her stealthily and insidiously. It would jump from her back to her pelvis over the course of any given day, from her hips to her belly, sometimes pausing everywhere in between. As a surgeon, I was accustomed to solutions and resented the treachery of this pain. Surgeons like to solve the problem at hand, and any ensuing problems, until the problems are gone. I can say with pride that most of the time we reach an end point where the child or young adult can go out into the world and thrive issue free.

But pain is still an insoluble issue, and was even more so fifteen years ago when I first met Victoria.

She had originally come to Dr. Randolph from West Virginia at age four with severe pain in her abdomen and pelvis. He had determined, after weeks of reading serpentine test results, that she had a very rare form of cancer, rhabdomyosarcoma, which manifested itself in her pelvic tissue. She was operated on for the first time at age five, and for several years after that she received intensive chemotherapy and radiation whenever the cancer reappeared.

Victoria had had numerous surgeries and rounds of chemo and radiation over the years, and now at last she wasn't just in remission, she was cancer free. I had inherited her case from Dr. Randolph when he left. After that first meeting, I saw Victoria every three or four months, and soon I, too, succumbed to her charms.

One time when I'd been working with her for about five years, I felt as if I could almost touch her pain, it was so present in the space between us. She was gritting her teeth, sitting rigidly, not wincing, but the pain permeated her body and her eyes. The radiation had affected the joints in her spine, and recently, after a series of CT scans, we had determined that the cancer treatment had actually stunted the growth of the spine's joints. While her vertebrae were growing normally, her joints were not. The net effect was a crushing pain in the nerves around the joints, where the growing bones were pressing. This caused her to walk gingerly, almost like an arthritic grandmother. As courageous as she was, she could not possibly hide that excruciating pain, and her nurses and I were devastated by our inability to help her.

My surgeon's impulse was to take a scalpel and cut here and there and everywhere and banish this girl's pain forever. But there was no clear way to help. Her pain popped up all over the place, like a villain in a horror movie. My only recourse, as I could not make her spinal joints grow, was to send her to yet another pain specialist who would prescribe yet another painkiller that would have a new set of side effects, which she would suffer through for a few years before developing resistance. Before long there would be no painkillers left to try.

I performed several surgeries after that to try to alleviate the bone pressure and remove the abdominal scar tissue that was contributing to her massive pain. The last surgery I performed was the riskiest. Her radiation treatments had left her with so much scar tissue in her abdominal organs that she had begun to experience severe blockages of her colon and bowels, given the proximity of the bowel to the pelvis. The radiation had affected tissues in the entire area, and the pain she felt as she struggled to pass her stool was almost unbearable.

The day we decided to operate, I touched a body more rigid and fraught with pain than any I had ever seen.

Victoria came in and sat down on my table, and my heart sank. She was in her late teens by now, but she appeared to be as frightened as a young child. She looked at me with tears in her eyes, and I felt them rising up to my eyes, too. I turned away and pretended to search for an instrument. This child was suffering in a way that I could not even imagine.

As she sat in the bland exam room, her colorful outfit brightening the space and my day, I tried to explain the risks of the procedure. Teens can tell when you are sugarcoating. Transparency and honesty are critical or you risk losing their trust. The same thing goes for parents, as back home kids will sense the gap if you tell them a different story.

Scar tissue is unpredictable, and I believed the operation ran a very high risk of further damaging her bowel. There is no abrupt point at which scar tissue stops and healthy tissue resumes, so the probability of having to cut or damage healthy tissue was far too high for my comfort level. My gut told me not to perform the operation. And I pretty clearly stated this to her.

But at one point in the exam, when she tried to find words to describe the severity of her pain, the tears welled up in her eyes again. I raised my hand. “I get it, I understand,” I said. “We’ll be a team. We’re going to try to help you through this.” We would operate the next day.

Should I have done it? Ethically, I am perplexed by this question to this day. I knew I could fix something, and it is in a surgeon’s DNA to go for the fix. But I could not fix the underlying problem. At best I could provide temporary relief, until the next piece of scar tissue twisted itself into a knot and caused her wrenching pain again. That could be next week or next year—or even the next day if we were not precise with our lasers.

That night I was despondent. I hugged my boys a little harder and longer than usual, hoping that their lot in life would never be as unfair as Victoria’s. I was about to perform a high-risk procedure in which the secondary objective, relieving pain, had become primary. We surgeons operate to perform and then measure a quantifiable fix. The tumor was there; the tumor is gone. The blood vessel was constricted; the blood vessel is open. The bone pressing on the nerve needs to be shaved; the nerve no longer feels pressed.

But in Victoria’s case, this procedure, ostensibly to unclog her bowel, was secondary to the objective that was now consuming her nurses, doctors, and me. No matter how hard we tried or how many fixes we successfully achieved, we could not alleviate her pain. And therefore we could not heal her.

I tried to rationalize the reason for the operation, as any surgeon would. We had to do it so she could process her body’s waste more effectively, and that was its own end. But the scar tissue was producing the pain that was devastating this beautiful child, and I knew we could never remove all the scar tissue in her pelvis without removing her pelvis itself.

I was doing something that Dr. Randolph had taught me to do: imagine this child's future. And I just could not imagine a future free of pain for her.

When I operated the next day, I tried too hard. I knew it was my job to cordon off a small part of my heart that my patients could never reach. But she had broken through every barrier I had been taught to put up. During the surgery, I operated out of anger. I saw the mangled bowel and scarred colon, and while I fixed the parts where blockages were occurring, I was distracted by what I knew would be the next spot where a blockage would occur, this year or next. I had prided myself on being the fixer of raw deals, but I couldn't fix Victoria, and I raged with a sense of responsibility for her future of pain. I couldn't help her break out of what her nurses had come to call her pain loop.

Victoria had great nurses who were as moved by her grace and guts as I was, but no one connected with her like Debbie Freiburg, a nurse in the oncology unit who became her primary advocate within the hospital. Debbie had become my main sounding board and chief consoler. But after this surgery, she raised with me an issue that I had not previously considered. Victoria was a young woman now. She was grappling with concerns about the appearance of her body after so many surgeries and treatments.

How could I not have been more sensitive to this? Why did I not think of taking additional care to make her feel more comfortable with herself, now that she was becoming a woman?

A more precise word than *pain* for this kind of chronic suffering, I discovered, is *anguish*. We surgeons so easily focus on physical pain because it is what we see. We can operate to alleviate it or prescribe medication to minimize it. But the psychological dimension of pain, and of being so persistently operated on as a child, was something I had failed to sufficiently focus on.

In my final years treating Victoria, we didn't have to deal with her abdominal issues because it was her spinal pain that became the constant source of difficulty. In one of our last visits, in 2005, she came into my office bent over and grimacing, her back twisted like an arthritic old woman's. She was in her twenties now. I asked her how her family was doing, and her grimace suddenly lifted. She looked up at me, blank-faced and startled, then shook her head and went back to grimacing. I realized later that I had distracted her momentarily from her pain.

Sometime later, to our delight, Victoria got married to a young man she had known in college. At some point her condition suddenly and steadily stabilized and the invasive surgeries finally ceased. Debbie kept me up on the gossip, and I was thrilled to learn that Victoria's marriage was fulfilling. I didn't see her for about five years. Then one morning a few years ago, Debbie walked into my office and sat in the chair on the opposite side of my desk. As soon as she said Victoria's name, I knew she was going to deliver bad news. Had the cancer popped up again in another form? After all, so many years of chemo and radiation at a young age can trigger cancer a few decades later.

As Debbie went on, I realized that it was more final than that. After a minute it finally hit me that Victoria had died. Debbie and I hugged each other, as doctors and nurses often do at times like this. We didn't know the circumstances of her passing; we never would. But the idea of never seeing her again was painful in its own way. For all her discomfort, she had brought us life.

Debbie and I went to Victoria's funeral in West Virginia, and during the service I pondered my role in this child's life. Had I preserved her so that she could suffer more? Did she die thinking that all those surgeries and treatments were just the adult world's way of perpetuating the bad hand she had been dealt at birth? Her death was a mystery, and I wanted it to stay that way. I wanted to hold on to a vision of her as alive and beautiful.

Pain, not cancer, had surely killed her, and so I believed medicine had failed her.

Before Victoria, when I had lost a patient, I had always been able to defend that supposedly impenetrable part of my heart. But the day I learned that she had died, something changed forever. Her passing would motivate me to mount an aggressive and systematic assault on pain. Her father still sends roses to Debbie and to Victoria's other nurses on her birthday. They are welcome reminders of his daughter's beauty and grace, but the best memorial to Victoria may someday soon be the near elimination of pain in pediatric medicine. She drives me, as exceptional patients drive so many doctors, to seek new solutions to seemingly intractable problems.

CHAPTER 16:

The Patient in the Data

For most of my time at Children's National, I thought only about surgery. I would drive to work each day, enter the building, focus on case after case, and go home to rest for a while, mulling over my cases, new techniques, or unforeseen complications. I never stopped to think about the dynamics of the hospital itself, or saw it as a sort of multicellular organism.

Dr. Anderson had sparked an interest in the functioning of the hospital when she challenged me to think differently about the needs and protocols of the NICU. I wouldn't say I suddenly aspired to a career in hospital administration, but I did develop an interest in the nitty-gritty of the hospital's functioning, in the different and disparate needs among its departments, and in its internal tensions.

One day Dr. Peter Holbrook, the chief medical officer (the doctor who manages all the other doctors), approached me with what he called an "opportunity." I had been an attending surgeon for well over a decade and was so busy and happy that as soon as I heard the word, I started thinking about how to dodge it.

"Kurt," he said, "I've got something for you."

That phrase usually prefaced an invitation to undertake an assignment that a more senior physician didn't want.

"Our quality control program," he said a bit cryptically. "I'd like you to work with a nurse on it. Kathy Gorman—she's the director of a new program to improve safety and hospital outcomes. Now we want to bring the doctors into it. See if you can make use of her findings to take her ideas to the next level."

It didn't sound too exciting. We use many euphemisms in medicine, particularly when we need to deliver bad news, and the term *quality control* struck me as a glaring euphemism for boredom. Whenever I heard the term as a young doctor, I assumed I could stop paying attention. Quality control was the realm of suits and calculators, not the way for a young doctor to pass his valuable time. I was hardly enthusiastic, but Dr. Holbrook's tone of voice told me that it wasn't an invitation so much as an assignment.

It took one meeting with Kathy Gorman to turn me around. Kathy had been an intensive care nurse for many years, and she had a great sense of the hospital's many complex points of vulnerability and weakness. Her data compilation and analyses focused on concerns like infection rates across different procedures, errors in the administration of medicine, and incomplete discharge instructions. She combined frontline nursing experience with data skills in a way that few medical professionals did, and her ability to blend care and metrics was something I had never before encountered. Where I had spent my career going from patient to patient, she saw typologies, trends, and patterns.

As a surgeon, I measured quality by specific outcomes—deaths, infections, prolonged hospital stays, successful interventions. As a surgical staff, we would analyze our cases on a weekly basis and look for variations and discrepancies from the norm. We would present our cases to one another at a peer review meeting called Morbidity and Mortality Conference (M&M for short, though it was nowhere near as cheerful as the candy). Here surgeons would challenge one another's judgment and technique when a patient died from complications. That was the general approach to "quality" throughout most surgical staffs nationwide—a transparent, case-based discussion about how to get better and avoid errors.

If an infection developed in a patient following surgery, we would look at the factors that might have contributed to the infection and assess any variations from the standard of practice. We would discuss whether the problem should be attributed to an individual surgeon or to the system of care, or if it had occurred because of the patient's disease or condition. If we determined that a surgical or planning error had occurred, Dr. Randolph would expect the surgeon or team to make the adjustments necessary to avoid that complication in the future. If we decided it was related to the patient's disease, then it was held up for collective consideration to prepare for when it might recur. If we felt it was a systemic issue, like the appropriate timing and dosage of antibiotic administration after an operation, we would establish new procedures.

For our first meeting, I had to venture down into the basement to Kathy's windowless office. The symbolism was not lost on me—she was doing something on the periphery that would require real innovative thinking and institutional creativity to bring into the mainstream.

"Where do we start?" I asked as I sat down, slightly dreading what was to come.

She pulled a huge binder full of protocols and notes off the shelf and handed it to me. "Here, this is the bible," she said, smiling mischievously. "Study this, and we'll be able to have a constructive conversation."

She walked me through a massive amount of data on physician performance, hospital indicators, and patient satisfaction. I was about to see the terms *correlation* and *causation* in a whole new way.

An hour into the meeting, I stopped her. "Why do they have you down here in the basement?" I said. "This is virtually the entire history of our hospital. Coming up with workable lessons out of all this data could transform the place."

"Try being a nurse for a day, and you'll see what it takes to get a doctor to listen," she said.

At our next meeting, Kathy explained that she and the chief nursing officer, Nellie Robinson, had been thinking about quality improvement for years but had not been able to get the medical leadership fully engaged. It was so caught up in the day-to-day running of the hospital that looking at the big picture was an interruption. There was always more urgent work to do. I remembered with some embarrassment my own reaction when Dr. Holbrook approached me.

Over the coming weeks, we focused on some obvious places where there was ample room for improvement. Her questions gripped me. Why did we have five different approaches to the same procedure? Why did some doctors order CT scans and some MRIs? Why did we treat asthma differently depending on which specialty was in charge? And couldn't we evaluate every procedure we performed? These sorts of questions were fundamental to improving the hospital's outcomes, but she just had not been able to build the momentum necessary to make quality improvement a functioning, standalone program.

Take the problem of appendicitis. The basic approach was to determine if a child had persistent right lower abdomen pain and tenderness. If so, we operated. If we learned during the operation that the child's appendix had burst, then we would treat her aggressively, giving triple antibiotics intravenously for seven to ten days until she was afebrile and had a normal white blood count. I was comfortable with this approach and had even standardized it with a number of local pediatricians. But each surgeon on staff had his or her own approach to appendicitis and his or her own protocol for antibiotics. Mine was one of many, and we all took that variability for granted.

Kathy decided we should start with appendectomies, this most obvious and frequent surgery—what we called appies—and standardize care.

We built a uniform program for appies and then analyzed a wide range of cases, including pneumonia, asthma, and sickle cell disease. We created a database that captured all the charges and orders electronically. We then analyzed the data by diagnosis, by surgeon, or by department to determine the optimal approach for each treatment.

Over the course of several months, we set up a system that allowed us to look at the outcomes of individual surgeons according to a number of measures—their rate of appendectomy for a ruptured appendix, their handling of antibiotics or imaging, and their rate of complications. By the end we could provide the surgery department with an analysis of the outcomes of individual surgeons and a broader departmental analysis. We found that among the six attending pediatric surgeons, there were six different ways of managing appendicitis. Likewise, there were multiple variations in the type of antibiotics and the length of treatment, the duration of hospitalization, and the criteria for discharging a patient. We were both thrilled and embarrassed by our discoveries.

One moment best revealed the difference between my perspective as a surgeon and Kathy's as a nurse. We were studying the length of hospital stays. Our data crunchers had produced an analysis of every stay of every patient over the past decade, broken down by condition or type of surgery. As Kathy and I sat side by side in front of spreadsheets in her basement office, I jumped on the issues that surgeons typically fixate on.

"Think about how much those extra days increase the risk of infection!" I said, "Think of how much it cost!"

An impish grin appeared on Kathy's face, and I knew I was about to get a different point of view. "Think of those extra days of missed school," she said. "Think of those parents having to burn through their vacation days to stay with their kid!"

Her immediate impulse was to analyze our discoveries through the lens of parents and patients. Like Dr. Anderson, Kathy Gorman was good at seeing data through the eyes of the people we were caring for. I was learning not only transformative lessons in data analysis but a new way of seeing the consequences of medical decisions.

When we extended our data analysis to imaging—CT scans and MRIs—we discovered a similar variability in orders and timing across different doctors for the same cases. Some surgeons insisted on an ultrasound or CT scan prior to surgery for a neck mass or a pleural effusion (buildup of fluid in the lungs), while others used no advanced imaging at all.

"We have to focus on the extra radiation risk some of these patients are being subjected to," Kathy said almost angrily.

I nodded and suggested we also consider the cost to families, as some surgeons had far lower overall billing on certain standard cases than others.

Our presentation did not go down well with the surgical team. We encountered resistance, skepticism, and irritation. A few doctors felt they were being micromanaged and insisted they knew what was best for their patients. But once everyone had had an opportunity to digest the data, most doctors began to appreciate the benefit of the changes that our analysis recommended. We agreed on the need to standardize treatments and procedures for a number of interventions, leaving leeway of course for specific circumstances and doctors' judgment calls.

Kathy was thrilled to see her work bear fruit, but she wasn't content to stop there. She suggested we tap into a network of thirty children's hospitals that had agreed to share data with one another through a centralized database. She wanted to see if the outcomes of hospitals across the country could be compared, in the hopes of defining the best practice for hundreds of procedures and treatments that were being performed daily at all these institutions. In addition to appendicitis, we did this analysis with sickle cell disease, asthma, bronchiolitis, and hernias.

We discovered a wide and chaotic range of protocols and results, and were able to identify the best practice for many problems. For example, the surgeons at Nicklaus Children's Hospital in Miami had developed a protocol to treat perforated appendicitis on an increasingly outpatient basis. Once the children became afebrile and had a normal white count after surgery, they were discharged. This was a radical approach, as most children's hospitals insisted on a seven-to-ten-day hospitalization for the delivery of intravenous antibiotics prior to discharge. The success of the Miami protocol made it clear that children could be discharged sooner, as the data revealed similar or lower complication rates.

We adopted the Miami protocol and quickly saw the advantages: shorter stays, less expense, and less family stress. In an era of advanced imaging, the age-old philosophy of erring on the side of surgery for appies was no longer necessary. We discovered that we could and should wait and began operating much less.

From 1999 until 2004, Kathy and I worked together to apply logic and statistics to a range of surgical and hospital-related procedures. Collaborating with her taught me that listening to and executing the ideas of nurses is fundamental to running a more efficient hospital. After all, nurses are the closest to patients, the most observant of hospital details, and the most intimately engaged in the nitty-gritty of care and results.

I also learned that data can be harnessed to improve practices and outcomes. Forced to grow out of my case-by-case tunnel vision, a world of opportunity opened up for pediatric medicine and for our hospital. Data analysis and application could transform outcomes, and a hospital that combined the art of patient care with the metrics of data analysis would marry the best of the past and the future.

CHAPTER 17:
The Mayor

Ever since my cancer surgery as a medical student, I have felt a special affinity with cancer patients who needed surgery. I gravitated toward those operations and developed a bit of a reputation for pediatric cancer surgery, particularly thyroid cancer. One of the deepest connections I have ever had with a cancer patient began when Casey showed up in my office around 2000. Two years earlier, when he was about twelve, he had hurt his leg in a soccer game. As his limp worsened and his discomfort persisted, his parents took him to an orthopedist. The pain seemed disproportionate to the severity of his injury. As is so often the case with bone cancer (where bone cells grow out of control and form tumors), the orthopedist was the gateway to the diagnosis. Looking at an X-ray of Casey's leg, he discovered not a hairline fracture in his femur but a baseball-size cyst. He sent Casey to an oncologist at Children's National, Dr. Nita Seibel, who ordered a biopsy. A few days later the pathologist determined that Casey's tumor was malignant. Dr. Seibel recommended chemotherapy followed by surgical removal of the cyst to attempt to preserve the limb and avoid an amputation. The initial results of the procedures were good, and the leg did not require amputation.

But by the time Casey was fourteen, his bone cancer had returned and so devoured his leg that our only recourse was amputation. In the two years since the soccer injury, he had undergone several rounds of chemotherapy.

Casey's cancer offered the perfect example of how biologically different kids are from adults. Cancers are usually much more aggressive in kids. Their bodies are growing at such a rapid rate—their cells differentiate and proliferate so quickly—that cancers move lightning fast. For the same reason, kids are much more responsive to aggressive cancer treatment. When Dr. Sidney Farber, the father of modern cancer treatment, first proved chemotherapy was effective, he used children with leukemia and tumors as his test cases. He began working with children, and was successful not least because of their heightened responsiveness to medications and interventions.

This biological willpower was good news for Casey. The bad news was that his cancer had already metastasized. Bone cancer, like many cancers, picks a reliable way to spread. More often than not, for reasons we don't yet understand, it metastasizes in the lungs. Once we spotted the cancer in Casey's leg, we knew the probability that it would manifest in his lungs was high. Dr. Seibel had done regular lung exams, and a couple of years after the second surgery, Casey and his mother showed up at my office with a CT scan of his lungs.

He was upbeat, almost carefree, so I was all the more shocked when I saw the images. He obviously knew what he had. I knew and respected Dr. Seibel and assumed that she had thoroughly communicated the extent of Casey's cancer to him.

"Looks like we get to spend some more time together, Dr. Newman," Casey said as I turned to look at him. "Doesn't that make you happy?"

Here he was, enjoying the day more than I or most of my colleagues were. You might write that off as this young man simply having been born with the happy gene. It was his nature, his predisposition—so much so that we had nicknamed him the Mayor—but that's not quite right. Casey wanted to thrive, and it was in his nature as a young person to satisfy that urge. Being so extroverted was just an overlay. He would become my model for the psychological willpower of children. The truth is, we overworry about our kids. Most of them are programmed to surmount obstacles so they can get out there and find their way. Sometimes all our worrying and meddling just get in the way.

Casey made a point of speaking with everyone he passed in the hall, from janitors to top docs. "How ya doin'?" he'd say, with a booming voice that made me think his vocal cords had overdeveloped. He'd pat fellow cancer patients on the shoulder and urge them to "keep fightin'." He was so forceful and consistent in his optimism that it had to be a life code for him. At the age of fourteen, he was looking fate in the eye and not flinching. He was clearly determined that we take the same approach.

Over the next few years, we performed four lung surgeries. Six months after the last one, Casey and his mother showed up with his worst CT scan yet. His lungs were riddled with spots. Had it been a child with less gumption, I probably would have spoken with Dr. Seibel about the futility of surgery at this stage. But not with Casey. I typically want to push kids, believing that their biology will withstand the harshest of treatments, but I had learned to balance this aggressiveness with an assessment of the child and the family. Are they on board? Do they really believe that this child can withstand the surgery? Is their hope grounded in reality?

A few years earlier we would have had to access Casey's lungs through his sternum—essentially cutting through his chest bone, as in open heart surgery. The pain and recuperation were brutal for children. But new techniques had been developed using video scopes, so we would now be able to make smaller incisions through each side of the chest. From there I'd actually use my fingers to remove each cancerous nodule, some the size of a marble, others as big as a Ping-Pong ball, and still others no larger than a little piece of grit. Imaging prior to surgery would reveal some of the nodules, but the hands-on technique was still the best way. I was going to spend a couple hours with my hands inside his collapsed lungs, looking for the devil's gold. Even in this age of advanced treatments and technology, the fingers were still the best tool for detecting tiny tumors. Casey was fortunate that the nodules had clustered at the bottom of his lungs and near the surface of the tissue there, rather than near the heart or deep in the lung tissue.

I felt I had to offer him the full prognosis. Again chemotherapy had not fully succeeded, and this was going to be his most significant intervention yet.

Our best-case scenario was that by removing the tumors, we'd give chemotherapy a better, and perhaps last, chance to eradicate the cancer. That was the optimist's view. With the larger nodules removed, the chemo would have less work to do and could focus more on his bones and any microscopic nodules in his lungs.

The realist's, or pessimist's, view was that even if we did successfully remove every nodule, numerous microscopic nodules would remain, impossible for me or anyone to locate by touch, and chemo would not be able to fully eradicate them.

The morning before the surgery I went to discuss the prognosis with Casey. As I walked into his room, before I had even sat down, he shouted "Newwwwwwman!" *Seinfeld* reruns were one of his favorite hospital viewing options, and Casey loved to mimic the show's signature jeer whenever he saw me. I lowered myself gently onto the corner of his bed. His cousin and parents sat in chairs nearby.

Casey took charge. "Look at this man's hands," he said, taking my left hand in his and lifting it up so one of his cousins could see. "You see these hands?"

The boy nodded.

"These are the hands of one of the greatest surgeons in the world," Casey continued, winking at me in exaggeration. "And they've been poking around inside me for years. He's now the chief of surgery. The chief!"

"Wow!" his cousin said.

"Look at them," Casey said. "He could've been a great piano player with these hands, and tomorrow they're going to be poking around inside me."

His cousin flashed me a look, equal parts disbelief and disgust.

I didn't correct Casey, because I wanted him to believe in those hands. In reality, I'd always considered myself in the middle of the pack in terms of surgical dexterity. My strong suit, which compensated for my average hands, was my practice of visualizing, planning, and executing the surgery. In that category, I prided myself on being near the top. I did correct him on my new title, for the technical term is surgeon in chief, and I had indeed at last inherited, on an interim basis, the job Dr. Randolph had held when I arrived at Children's National twenty years prior. It was now 2003, and I couldn't help but think how much Dr. Randolph would have loved interacting with a patient as vital as Casey.

But Casey had disarmed me, too. I'd rehearsed what I thought would be a hard conversation, and in a matter of minutes he'd undermined my script. He was also, shrewdly, motivating me. Here was this savvy kid building up my surgeon-size ego the day before I was about to cut into him. I knew what he was up to, but it still worked. Perhaps because he was such a sports fan, Casey understood the power of motivation. He was like the best coaches, who are master motivators. With his cousin as our audience, he'd pumped me up to operate as no one had ever done before.

I decided not to even broach the risks and downside of the surgery, as we surgeons are obligated to do. He didn't want to hear it. He was so insistent on optimism that I knew I could dispense with medical formalities.

I'd walked into his room dreading the conversation and somehow managed to leave on an upbeat note.

The next day during surgery, as I was probing Casey's lungs with my fingers and extracting nodule after nodule, I couldn't help but think of how he had praised my hands. I knew I was performing at the level he'd set for me. He had done it on purpose, holding my hands up to motivate me. What a master, I thought.

When we'd removed every nodule that had shown up as a spot on the CT scan, I probed both lungs with my fingertips, hoping against hope that those dreaded microscopic tumors might magically reveal themselves. I focused more intensely than I ever have in my life, sometimes closing my eyes and directing all my brainpower toward the sensations in my fingertips. I wanted my hands to be as good as he'd said they were.

Throughout the next year, after Casey recovered, many of us talked about him at random moments. People in pediatrics routinely attach to patients and enjoy their company, though to see them again in the hospital is the last thing we want. That paradox of our profession confounds me. Kids like Casey make me not only a better surgeon but also a better father and colleague. His optimism—defiant, natural, and unceasing—had rubbed off on me. I found myself being more encouraging of my own sons, urging them to see the bright side of any struggle or fear.

Occasionally, when looking at a calendar, I'd realize that I was counting the days and weeks since Casey's surgery—and I wasn't the only one. Many of his caretakers would regularly comment on how many days or months it had been since we last took orders from the Mayor. On his fifteenth birthday, several doctors and nurses and I noted it as we passed each other in the halls.

But then about three months after his birthday, Dr. Seibel called me, and I knew what it meant. The cancer had gone wildfire again and was all over Casey's lungs. I thought back to the last surgery, how I had probed every inch of his lungs for nodules. I hung up the phone and rubbed my face. I felt as if my supposedly magical fingers had been revealed as duds.

After we subjected Casey to a battery of CT scans and blood work, Dr. Seibel recommended that we forgo further treatment and simply focus on improving the quality of his remaining life. One afternoon in the fall of 2006, I sat in my office and struggled to find some way to resist. I looked up at his CT scan: tumor nodules had reappeared throughout his lungs, triple the number we'd seen and removed in his last operation. The cancer was back in his bones, too. I knew that when I went upstairs to discuss the situation with Casey, I'd face his boundless, aggressive optimism, so I rehearsed ways to convince him that this time was different. This time we were at the end of the line. Ask yourself: How would you say this to a teenager, especially one who is preternaturally incapable of believing it?

I swallowed, pushed myself out of my chair, and began what felt like a death march. As Dr. Seibel and I walked to his room, it was getting dark outside. I knew I had to take control of the conversation from the get-go and cut Casey off if he began talking. This time I couldn't let him commandeer the tone and agenda.

In his previous stay, he'd looked askance at the huge animal murals we'd painted in the patients' rooms and declared that he'd outgrown the childish themes and bright colors. We needed, he claimed, a ward just for teenagers who drove pickup trucks, like him. With this in mind, upon walking into this room, I registered the big cow painted on the wall at the foot of his bed. It was oversize and out of proportion to the surrounding farm animals. It had big black spots that looked like a bad modern painting.

I smiled at Casey but tried to use body language to forecast my message, not even chuckling at my "Newwwwwwman!"

I sat in one of the hospital chairs, its back so straight I felt forced to lean forward. I looked at him and saw the softest, most receptive face I've ever seen in an adolescent. He'd given me liberty to say what I needed to say.

"Another operation is not going to help you, Mr. Mayor," I said. "We won't be able to remove the tumors. There are too many, and they're too deep, and we'd be just putting you through a lot of unnecessary pain. If there were any chance of helping you, I'd do it, you know that, but I just can't see this helping you at all."

Dr. Seibel covered for me as I ran out of words. "We'll see if there's any other therapy that might help, anything experimental," she said.

Casey didn't blink. He looked at Dr. Seibel, then at me, calmly.

"I hear you guys loud and clear," he said. "But why did you have to pick my final visit here to put me in the room with the stupid cow looking at me all night?"

He succumbed to his cancer about six months later.

Casey wasn't simply a lesson in sentiment or character for us. Because he lived optimistically and positively to the end, he was a challenge to us about how to practice pediatric medicine and especially pediatric oncology. His life, and his valiant end, would become a long pep talk for me and my team as, several years later, we set about reinventing the ways our society treats sick and ailing children.

Donors give hospitals millions of dollars and get their names on halls and wings; researchers discover genetic secrets that could put them in the

Nobel Prize league; doctors make technical innovations that will be studied in medical schools for years. But every once in a while, the legacy of a kid like Casey surpasses all those credentials. We still celebrate his birthday every year at the hospital. But, more profoundly, his ghost comes back to give us those pep talks.

What Casey taught me, his part-time surgeon and the full-time butt of his jokes, was that professional doctors and nurses are fundamentally vulnerable and easily moved by the sort of heroic grandeur that our patients can display. Put more simply, Casey made us feel better about ourselves and our work. He made us feel better about life.

The day he died, I knew we had to do more. I cherished the amazingly responsive biology of kids and their stunning mental toughness, but the pain many of them had to go through seemed insulting. Casey had been my favorite patient, not just for his personality and charisma but because his cancer had forced me to work with people in other fields—Dr. Seibel, nurses, pain management folks, orthopedists—to find a comprehensive solution.

Most of all I knew there had to be a way to treat pediatric cancer as distinct from adult cancer, to use imaging, chemotherapy, and radiation in a more precise fashion while attacking the genetic origins of the disease more aggressively and creatively. I had a hunch that children would be the place where we would first begin to defeat cancer. In some forms of pediatric leukemia, the success rates of targeted molecular treatments were skyrocketing. Children and adolescents deserved to be more of a priority in cancer research, not only because they have a longer life ahead of them but also because they would be more responsive patients, given their biological and psychological resilience.

The memories of Casey and Victoria would spur me to try not only to defeat pain and cancer but to separate them. I wanted to be able to treat cancer in children in a way that spared them the pain they suffered as much from their therapies as from the disease. A charismatic fellow named Joe Robert, one-quarter crazy and three-quarters visionary, would show us how to turn this inspiration into a tangible, and successful, medical program.

CHAPTER 18:
A Man with a Plan

When I first started working for Dr. Randolph, the thrill of the start-up atmosphere at Children's National appealed to the young man I was. It energized me not only to be doing good but to be an outsider, too. As I matured, my beliefs about pediatric health care grew more nuanced and empirical. Babies whom I had operated on were coming back as thriving children. Adolescents who had been regular visitors to our clinics were showing up with their own children for exams and treatments. These kids we had helped became adults and had kids of their own who sometimes needed our help, too. The cycle of life was gratifying and beautiful. I was also learning more about the business side of health care, and I could see the folly of dedicating billions of dollars to adult medicine when investment in children clearly provided more long-term bang for the buck. But ailing children don't have well-funded lobbies in Washington advocating for them. They don't tend to recover from a devastating illness and set up nonprofits to obliterate it. Children don't court the media and establish support groups.

I had seen some progress nationally as I made my way through my career. Pediatric medicine—and pediatric surgery in particular—gained clout in medical schools and health systems. There were more pediatric centers embedded in adult hospitals, although the number of independent children's hospitals had plateaued around thirty. But the outlook, the social vision, was still dreadfully skewed toward investment in adult research and care, and it bugged me and my old mentor that his "frogs" were still not receiving the priority at the policy and philanthropic level that they deserved.

"It will happen," I'd tell Kathy Gorman and other colleagues halfheartedly. But I didn't really believe the overall system would change. The adults who had the power were always going to invest in the diseases that affected them and that promised more lucrative returns on investment.

That was just one pediatric surgeon's opinion, and I encountered little to challenge it until I met a local business leader in a massive, smoke-filled room full of loud, rowdy men who were puffing cigars and drinking scotch. I had come of age under the tutelage of the best pediatric specialist I could imagine; now I was about to undergo a crash course in how to apply Dr. Randolph's lessons on a bigger stage.

The first time I attended the legendary Washington philanthropic event called Fight Night in the late 1990s, I was stunned—not by the sight of men beating each other up in the name of the charity Fight for Children, but rather by the swagger of the event's host, a D.C. business legend named Joe Robert. Fight Night was one of the biggest charity events in the capital. Joe had harnessed his mix of bravado and generosity to persuade people to open up their wallets and support children. Joe, as I would soon learn, was a natural motivator.

Held in the massive main ballroom of the Washington Hilton, the event was far removed from the stately diplomatic dinners in nearby Embassy Row. The main course was a thick steak. There was lots of loud music—Sinatra, of course—but no dancing because it was a "sans spouse" event. In fact, it was one of the most politically incorrect events in Washington, but it raised tens of millions of dollars over the years for local charities. That excuse worked well enough to get scores of wives in the area to permit their husbands to act like cavemen for a night.

Joe's favorite philanthropic focus was to bring better educational opportunities to underprivileged kids in Washington, D.C. He grew up in a family that didn't have a lot of money and became part of the financial elite not through bloodlines or connections but through guts and grit. He worked his way up from selling condos to mastering the mortgage security business, and in the process he became a famous, and occasionally infamous, jet-setting multimillionaire. Now his main thrill in life was to give kids from "the streets" a chance to make it, too. His other big interest was children's health, and he had long been a strong supporter of Children's National. He also happened to have been an amateur Golden Gloves boxer, and the idea of combining pugilism and philanthropy surely was an American original. He created an endowed professorship called the Fight for Children Chair of Pediatrics, which supported many research initiatives.

At the time I was a full member of the surgical staff but far from a big shot. I received an invitation to fill out a table and provide a little medical credibility to the group. Unsure what I was getting into, I'd had my tuxedo dry-cleaned, but I could have saved myself a few bucks. At the evening's end, I had to enter my house through the back door and take off my tuxedo in the garage because it had absorbed so much cigar smoke. In fact, it took several days to get rid of the odor.

Joe's powerful handshake that night was part electroshock, part hand-hug, part declaration of a ferocious passion for life. In a city known for the transience and decorum of its so-called elite, Joe was a proud and defiant showman. In a town known for politics, he was anything but politic.

I enjoyed my first Fight Night, but I felt tired and baffled by this hurricane of a man upon whom so much of what we did at the hospital depended. I felt the same sort of dislocation that I had felt when I started my work at Harvard. And yet I knew I had to take a deep breath and adjust to this sort of bravado, for watching Dr. Randolph had taught me just how much philanthropy meant to a relatively impoverished hospital like Children's. As the financial challenges at the hospital and in medicine in general increased, he had spent more and more time off-site at fund-raisers for the surgery department. He never complained, but I could tell he felt that every minute spent away from surgery was a waste of time.

All this came back to me a few years later, when I found myself sitting in an examination room studying the chest of a nineteen-year-old muscular college student named Joey. As surgeons, we tend to latch on to certain procedures, so that they become favorites. The reasons are hard to explain. Perhaps we have had experience with the procedure ourselves, or perhaps it presents a specific technical challenge or artistry. Perhaps a mentor challenged us with it, or perhaps we had early success with it. Why do some people like and excel at baseball and others at gymnastics or tennis? Whatever the reason, most surgeons will acknowledge that certain operations just click and become favorites.

For me, one of those procedures was the repair of *pectus excavatum* and *pectus carinatum*, congenital abnormalities of the chest wall. *Pectus excavatum*—we saw a case of it in Chapter 6—is marked by a sunken chest. The ribs and cartilages are structurally out of alignment, creating a major cosmetic and structural abnormality of the anterior chest wall. *Pectus carinatum* is the opposite: the ribs, cartilages, and sternum protrude to make the chest bow outward, becoming more pronounced in the teenage years. Both conditions, as they become more apparent, can trigger psychological consequences for teenagers, especially self-esteem issues.

Joey had come alone to see me—he could do so at his age without parental consent—to discuss his *pectus carinatum*. I examined him, told him quite explicitly about the problem, and discussed the steps required to fix it. It would entail a major operation to radically change his ribs and the contours of the chest wall. It would mean removing some of the cartilage, repositioning the sternum, and then holding it in place with one or two temporary titanium bars. Because he was older and much of the cartilage had become more calcified, it would require heavy-duty cutting and therefore the recovery would be fairly long and painful.

He hesitated for a second when I asked him to take off his shirt so I could examine him. But as he asked me about the possible complications of the procedure, and its risks and benefits, I was impressed by his maturity. "Look, this is gonna be a tough procedure, but we'll be in it together and you'll come out looking really good," I said.

"Let me think about it, and I'll let you know next week," he said.

That afternoon a fellow surgeon asked me how my meeting had gone with Joe Robert's son. It wasn't until then that I put the two together: Joey Robert was Joe Robert's son!

I thought through everything I had told him, worrying that his report back to his father would raise a flag. I fixated on the word *stigma*. I had said to him, "This condition is really just a stigma, and that's unfortunate, but surgery will eliminate that feeling from your life."

Had I misspoken? Had I used too strong a word?

Pediatric surgeons loathe the idea of stigmas, as well as the teasing and bullying that so many children endure simply because they have the misfortune to be born or to develop a disease, atypical condition, or deformity. I knew I would have to negotiate a complicated father, but I told myself that so far I had done the right thing.

A week or so later, I got the call I had been fearing. Joe Robert said he had done some research on me and understood that I had developed a focus on this specific condition. He wanted to know what my recommendation was. Slightly taken aback, I repeated my recommendation and plan. When I hung up, I put certain clues together and realized Joey had given his father a full report. Joe had just wanted to hear the recommendation from the horse's mouth.

I was sure Joey had made a firm decision to change the way people saw him, and the way he saw himself. But many teenagers live in their parents' shadows or in fear of them. As much as I had learned to advocate for parental involvement with the medical team, I had also refined my antennae for meddling, manipulative, and domineering parents. I was suspicious, given Joe Robert's powerful demeanor and reputation, that he might be all three.

Joey came back a few weeks later, alone again, and told me it was a go. He seemed lighter and happier already. He understood that he was in for a six-hour operation, that we were going to break a bunch of bones in his chest and insert a steel bar, and that the recovery would be slow and painful. At the end of our meeting, he looked me in the eyes and extended his hand. I shook it, remembering the handshake his father had given me at Fight Night.

"You're going to be fine," I said. "No matter what it takes, we're going to do this well and get you through it."

The surgery went well, and when I visited Joey in the recovery room, his father was sitting with him. Joe Robert stood up calmly, extended his hand, and smiled. He seemed less gregarious, and the contrast unnerved me.

Then Joey, in his anesthetized haze, managed to look down at his chest and see its new contour. He raised both hands slightly and gave me a double thumbs-up.

During Joey's recovery, I met a new Joe Robert. He clearly savored caring for his son. He spoke to me three or four times a day. He spent the ten-day postoperative course at his son's bedside, often sleeping in the room at night with him. Joey was in significant pain and was hooked up to a couple of IVs. His father took to managing his vast business empire from the hospital chair, using an outsize cellphone to make calls all over the world. But he didn't seem outsize himself; he wasn't on his home turf and seemed very human compared with the man I had met at Fight Night.

As the days went on, Fight Night Joe slowly returned. He grew agitated by some of the care being given to his son and by the noise and the interruptions of Joey's sleep. Depending on his needs and mood, he grilled me, or enlightened me, or ordered me. Many doctors grow frustrated by this sort of situation—the surgery goes well, but then things we can't control undermine the sense of success.

Early one morning I walked in, and he promptly told me how uncomfortable the bed and the couch in the room were. "Last night you know what I did?" he asked. "I laid a blanket on the floor and slept there. I slept better." He had stayed at some of the finest hotels in the world, he told me, and they had all sorts of wonderful extravagant comforts, but they did not cost as much as the thousand dollars a night that we were charging him to sleep on the floor.

Part of me was irritated by this rich guy complaining about his discomfort. I had seen thousands of parents suffer through thick and thin for their child. A few had complained, often jokingly, about the poor sleeping conditions. *We aren't a luxury hotel,* I wanted to say to Joe, *and the kids' beds are what matter,* though I couldn't summon the nerve to say it out loud.

A few days later I walked in to check on Joey, but his father cut me off before I could get a word in. "In no hotel room in the world, not even the dirtiest fleabag of a place, would I ever be awakened six times a night," he said.

I nodded and went to walk around him to get to his son, but his body blocked my path.

"Joe, look, I'm just a surgeon," I said. "I will register your complaints, but I want to take care of your son. I can't change the system."

"Bullshit!" he said.

I stepped back.

His face reddened, and he stepped toward me. "You think I care if they wake me up?" he asked angrily. "I don't sleep more than five hours a night wherever I am. Don't need it. But my son right now needs it. You know what? I walked up and down these halls last night. You have some beautiful kids here. Beautiful families. They bring tears to my eyes, their love and devotion. But your staff and your machines are waking them up over and over, all night long. I'm no doctor, but isn't it during sleep that a child heals? Isn't that when a child grows? Or is that an old wives' tale?"

He stopped, shook his head, and stepped aside.

I was rattled but still wanted to examine Joey. As I approached him, I noticed he was blushing. "How are you feeling this morning?" I asked.

He looked down at his chest: the bandage was now off. Despite the single scar, which we were treating, too, his chest was flat and rounded.

"Looking good," I said, extra loud so his father would hear. "Looking good!"

On my last visit before Joey's discharge, his father was sitting in his chair, talking on his cellphone. He spotted me. I tried to avoid eye contact with him as I walked over to Joey's bed.

"I'll call you right back," I heard him say as he clicked off the phone.

"The food in this joint wouldn't get even half a star in a *Washington Post* review," he said to me. "But it sure as hell costs more than any five-star restaurant."

I didn't respond. I examined Joey, signed the discharge papers with a little excess flair, and shook Joey's hand. "You're going to be the hit of the beach this summer," I told him.

He smiled broadly.

His father came over to the bed, beaming, and I shook his hand, too.

"I'll see you soon," he said. "Good work. But we're going to make some changes here. I'll give you a call soon."

A few weeks after Joey was discharged, I received a call asking me to meet with Joe Robert at his office in northern Virginia. I knew I was not the guy for this, and I called Dr. Randolph in Nashville to discuss my dilemma, as I still occasionally did when I was up against a tough one.

"We've got to tell our story well for the sake of the children," Dr. Randolph said. "He wants you to tell our story better. If he picked you, he picked you. He's got a reason. Remember when I told you, back when I offered you the job, you've got to be a community doctor? Well, that means working with rich guys, too. They keep us going. Go out there and learn from him."

He paused, and I envisioned him cradling the phone a little closer. "And bring back a check, too!" he said with a laugh.

Joe's office was in a glass skyscraper near Tysons Corner, next door to a Ritz-Carlton Hotel. It was on one of the top floors and had a commanding view of northern Virginia and, in the distance, the Washington, D.C., skyline. Charts and wallboards with fancy algorithms covered the walls. Joe's assistants disarmed me with their hospitality, which seemed a little at odds with the high-tech skyscraper offices.

I fully expected to hear some criticisms, and when Joe started our discussion by saying that after spending time at Children's, he knew we needed help, my immediate thought was that I was going to get in trouble with the hospital administration.

But he quickly shifted direction. "I'm the guy who's going to help you achieve what you can be," he said. "We'll fix this place together. You guys have the makings of the best pediatric surgery center in the world. A lot of the pieces are in place. Now we'll find the rest of them and build a program that will be a model for caring for kids for the next century."

Joe thought that by investing in the facilities and the patient experience, we could make major advances in results. This meant not only creating new operating rooms to attract the best surgeons and new waiting and recovery rooms for families, but also taking a deep look at the comprehensive experience of patients and parents in the hospital and on the floors. Sleep, food quality, Internet access—he was talking about the nitty-gritty of hospital life and tying that experience to overall clinical success.

We shouldn't separate the medical experience from a more holistic experience that would promote healing, he riffed. He envisioned private rooms for every patient so they could heal with their families in relative peace. He urged us to humanize the waiting rooms, because people spend time there in difficult and pressurized circumstances. He said we should consider the parents' professional and emotional needs and provide comfortable beds and chairs for them, as well as washing machines and showers. We should offer high-speed Internet access and rooms for spiritual contemplation. He urged us to bring more light and art and music into the patient experience. He felt our Child Life program, run by a small group of psychologists and social workers who sought to help children maintain a sense of fun and ritual during treatment, should be expanded.

"Holistic," he kept saying. I was shocked. He was sounding awfully New Age for a hard-charging, cigar-smoking businessman. "You are taking me by surprise," I said.

"Why, do I need to be more of a jerk? You like me better that way?"

It was hard to know how to answer.

"Look, you saw me at my worst, just like you see every parent in those circumstances," he said. "I was exhausted. I have a complicated family life. I love my son more than anything, and seeing him in pain kills me. It kills me. But you guys fixed that. You gave him a new sense of self in a couple of weeks. You've got me. You've got me forever. Now use me. Let's do something big."

He had even dug into my field of surgery. Now he asked me about the types of operating rooms and technology we used. He knew we were somewhat limited by our capital and couldn't provide operating rooms for every specialty, but he wanted us not only to expand the operating rooms' capacity and number but to dedicate specific ones to certain specialties, like neurosurgery and cardiac surgery.

This discussion, and a few more like it in which I primarily listened, soon led to a major gift to Children's National to create the Joseph E. Robert, Jr., Center for Surgical Care. From 2000 to 2006, we planned and raised money for it, then kicked off the construction phase. Over the course of that time I became the chief of surgery. It was an honor to hold Dr. Randolph's old job, and it gave me a platform from which to implement the things I was learning from Joe. It had been my ambition to be a surgeon in chief somewhere. Typically you have to move elsewhere to rise, so to hold the job at my own hospital was doubly rewarding.

My collaboration with Joe Robert became the most fulfilling aspect of my tenure at Children's National. We were going to transform the spaces where I had been working for twenty years, and memories of the difficult operations and camaraderie I had experienced on the old operating rooms filled my head. We spent months poring over blueprints and technology options, and it was fun to see doctors, nurses, and architects and engineers collaborate on behalf of kids. I spent hours trying to decide on the right lights for the OR, analyzing the layouts of the booms from which the new equipment would hang, selecting video and computer technology to be integrated, and then of course budgeting it all.

On the day of the public announcement, we all wore construction hats, and I felt just a little out of place with the construction guys all around. But

Joe was right at home, directing the excavation guys and telling the laborers and foremen what types of surgeries would be taking place in these future operating rooms. He led a capital campaign with another great Washington philanthropist, Diana Goldberg, and contributed $25 million of his own money to it. Their success set the stage for a $500 million campaign, which at that time was the largest amount ever raised for a children's hospital.

This investment allowed us to build a set of new operating rooms with the latest surgical technology. The surgeons would have operating rooms dedicated to their specialties—heart surgeons had their own advanced technology; eye surgeons had permanent microscopes installed in their OR; neurosurgeons had MRI machines for intraoperative MRI imaging. We were the talk of the pediatric surgery world, and the résumés of world-class surgeons and anesthesiologists arrived from around the globe.

More important, Joe's focus on the patient experience bore dividends and even changed my view of the surgical experience for children. He made me see more clearly that success wasn't just about flawless surgical procedure—we should strive for the same high standards in considering the experience of the child and the parent before and after surgery. Joe honed in on seemingly small issues like the number of times a patient might be awakened during the night to be checked on by nurses, the noise levels on the floors, the quality of the food and beds, and other basic comforts that could promote healing. He was a massive champion of paying attention to details. His personal drive and attention to detail galvanized an effort to improve every aspect of the surgical experience. We brought the specifics—the technology, the layout, the types of equipment, the requirements of anesthesiologists and nurses—and he breathed life into ideas about pediatric care that had been brewing for decades at Children's National but had never quite taken hold.

The medical-industrial complex was growing inexorably, and that was the biggest impediment to transforming the hospital. At some point in the 1990s, insurance companies became our real antagonists, imposing limits and controls on our actions in order to decrease costs and maximize profits.

Medicine had become, with swift and devastating finality, all about money. This was true even of pediatric medicine. I sometimes felt as if it happened overnight. Most of us had gone into this field to earn a good living, to do what we loved, and above all to help children. We had kept our heads down and worked hard for our patients, only to discover that we had somehow become part of a massive financial and administrative bureaucracy.

I accepted the reality of our need for philanthropists like Joe Robert, just as I remained devoted to the many financially challenged parents who loved their children as much as Joe loved Joey. But to break new ground and truly innovate, we had to fight money with money, and Joe made for a great financial field general.

Meanwhile Joey was thrilled with the outcome of his surgery. A year after the operation, he came to me and asked for medical clearance to hike the Appalachian Trail. Although he still had the bar in his chest, I thought it would be a great opportunity for him to meet such a tough challenge. Soon after that we determined that his healing was complete and we removed the bar. In 2002 he decided to join the Marine Corps but needed another medical clearance to do so.

It was a tricky proposition. I sensed that Joe Robert was secretly hoping I would not sign that permission form. But I could think of no medical reason why Joey could not pursue his dream. I sat there, the form in front of me on my desk. Joey looked at me with his father's intensity. I picked up a pen, held it over the page for a moment, and signed the form.

The next day I received a phone call from his father. "How could you sign a paper to put my son in harm's way?" the voice boomed.

But I soon realized, to my relief, that he was putting on an act.

"I am so proud of this guy," he said. "My son is going to be a Marine!"

He would go on to serve a tour of duty in Iraq as a member of an elite special forces unit. I saw him in uniform several years later at a ceremony in Quantico, and I could not stop thinking this young man might have helped me more than I had helped him. Dr. Randolph taught us to pay no heed to the official boundaries and protocols of medicine. He encouraged us to become friends with mothers and fathers and our patients. In this case, I found a mentor as different from Dr. Randolph as I could ever have imagined, but he was the perfect person to help me bring new ideas about pediatric care into practice.

Over the next few years, we constructed that state-of-the-art operating room for neurosurgery with a built-in MRI. Instead of having to close a patient's skull midsurgery and wheel them over to radiology for a scan, neurosurgeons could now get real-time scans during their operations to make sure they had removed every last piece of a tumor. We recruited a new chief of general surgery, Dr. Tony Sandler, a nationally renowned pediatric surgeon who was leading the fight to cure certain forms of cancer by harnessing the body's immune system. And we recruited Dr. Richard Jonas, a world leader in congenital heart surgery, who advocated correcting heart defects in infants and newborns instead of waiting until later in childhood.

October is my favorite month in Washington—warm but not too hot, leaves on full display but not yet fallen from the trees. Not long after Columbus Day in 2007, I was full of energy and ideas when Joe summoned me out to his massive house in Virginia for what I thought would be a strategy session. I prepared a presentation for him on the surgery department, focused on local and regional growth. When I arrived, I launched right in. Joe listened intently at first, but after a little while he started to fidget. Then he abruptly raised his hand, signaling for me to stop.

"We're going to take it even further, make it even bigger," he said. "You're thinking too small. You're not just a local hospital, or a regional hospital, or a resource for the kids and other hospitals in this area. You need to be thinking about becoming the best in the nation or in the world. You have to expand your vistas and recruit national and international superstars and attract patients from across the country and around the world for your programs. And most of all, you've got to create new things. Monetize them.

You know what that means? It means make money off them. New surgical tools. Vaccines. Cures!"

This guy never quit. But now, as surgeon in chief, I no longer felt threatened by his demands.

I spent several weeks sketching a new plan for innovation and went back out to him with a three-page outline. We sat at a table in front of his big fireplace and ate a breakfast of fresh-squeezed orange juice and organic cereal.

As I began sharing the plan with him, he again stopped me cold. "This is not what I have in mind," he said flatly. "You're just nickel-and-diming improvements here, adding a surgeon here or a surgeon there, or an anesthesiologist or a small program, but it's not what I had in mind. I want you to think about what it's like for a child to have had surgery ten or fifteen years from now. What would it take to radically change that experience? To transform it? What are the tools of the future? Can you invent new ones? And what kinds of patents could grow out of that? How do you make this center run like a business that not only provides the best services but creates medical advances that we can bring to the marketplace?"

I was getting a sense of how Joe worked: push, accomplish, and then push some more. But I also realized something more fundamental. Joe could be the sort of lobbyist children were missing; he could become their version of the AARP. He had money, he had friends with money, and he could raise even more.

After speaking with surgeons and scientists at other institutions around the country, I drafted a plan with more daring innovation—not just in surgery but in postop care, pain management, robotics, and imaging—as its core. No one inside medicine thought about innovation the way Joe did. His efforts at Children's were becoming the perfect prototype for a joint business-school–medical-school curriculum. A hospital had to run as a business, he understood, and yet it needed philanthropy to build the kinds of programs that it could never sustain as a business. I was out of my league but learning quickly and beginning to enjoy the ride.

The next time I went out to see him, he focused on how we could upend the medical supply chain so that we were no longer simply taking things that worked in adults and modifying them for children. The system always worked backward from what adults needed and used. Whether it was a pain score or a scalpel, a mask or a medication, kids traditionally got hand-me-downs from the world of adult medicine.

What emerged from Joe's tutorial was a vision of an institute of pediatric surgical innovation comprised of surgeons, anesthesiologists, bioengineers, educators, scientists, and radiologists brought together to constantly develop the new tools, techniques, and partnerships required to transform pediatrics. I recruited surgeons, scientists, imaging specialists, and bioengineers from Children's National to help write the final version of the proposal that had as its mantra "to make surgery for children more precise, less invasive, and pain-free." With children like Victoria and Casey still fresh in our minds and hearts, we created a rudimentary business plan, and I finally felt ready to go back to Joe for his review. We would try to understand the biology of pain, how it worked for children, and would then tailor the medications and treatments specifically to children's biology and psychology. As for surgical tools, we would construct a biomechanics lab to invent our own.

As Joe reviewed the proposal, he nodded and said, "Now, this is what I had in mind." I was hugely relieved. I had never wanted to impress a colleague or med school professor as much as I wanted to impress this guy. Finally we had done it. But then he stood up and started spinning around for about twenty seconds. He stopped, looked me hard in the eyes, and said, "Next step!"

He asked me to come back with a more formal business plan and proposal with numbers—hard, cold dollars—as its foundation.

We had many considerations to bring together: space for a home for the institute; the types of doctors and scientists required, and their salaries; the lab for innovations in tools and techniques. It took us a while to get the numbers to make sense, but in the end we found the right businesspeople on our board and in our community to craft a proposal precisely calculated at $100 million. This would cover the bricks and mortar, the brainpower, and the ongoing investigations, experiments, and intellectual laboratories. One night, working very late on the final review of this document, I realized Joe was giving me and my team a chance to raise pediatric medicine to the level of adult medicine—to give kids a creative spotlight right here in the nation's capital. At last we would have a shot at shifting the debate about where to invest our health care dollars and energies. Joe understood the return on investment, or ROI in business terms, offered by shifting our spending to the developing child. He looked at it as a societal investment in the untapped potential of children who had their entire lives ahead of them. He wanted to detect, prevent, and solve health problems at an early stage, rather than curing them after the fact or handling issues that developed after lifelong chronic diseases.

Soon I made the trek out to Joe's house in Virginia again, this time with Pam King Sams, the head of our foundation. He read the proposal in silence for half an hour while we waited. Finally, he raised his head and smiled gently—something I had never seen him do.

"The timing is perfect," he said. "I am going to restructure my company, and I will use some of the profits from selling a portion of it to fund this institute."

We agreed to call the venture the Institute for Pediatric Surgical Innovation. This champion capitalist was preparing to make the investment of his life. Over the years, I had met several people with Joe's kind of wealth, and many had given generously to the hospital, but Joe wasn't just going to give us a slice off the top. He was actually going to cut into his personal wealth. His skin, as he loved to say, was in the game.

But it was now the fall of 2008. The economy was going into free fall, and Joe's business, like almost everyone else's, came under an assault the likes of which he had never seen. The value of his company plummeted. He kept telling me not to worry; he was confident he'd come out strong on the other side of the crisis. At the hospital, the team I had assembled to present the project to various other donors and groups shuffled nervously. Months went by, and the news from Wall Street kept worsening. We hadn't put our fund-raising campaign on hold, but giving had dried up across many philanthropic endeavors. But Joe kept saying I should stick with him, and he never altered his commitment or his optimism despite his company's struggles.

Seven or eight months later I was mowing my lawn on a summer day when I received a call from Joe and his chief of staff, Daniel Radek, to tell me that they were planning a trip to the Middle East and wondered whether I had any of the slick proposal books about the institute. I had no idea where he was headed or what he was going to do with the books, but I figured whatever he had in mind, it could only help.

Several weeks later the phone rang the middle of the night. This type of call usually meant an urgent surgery, but this time it was Joe.

"Kurt," he said, "I'm over here. I was just talking with these people, and they're going to do it. They're going to do the whole thing."

"Joe," I said sleepily but politely, "where are you? Who is going to do what?"

"I'm in Abu Dhabi, Kurt," he said, as if it were the most natural place in the world for him to be. "I was meeting at the palace with the Crown Prince Sheikh Mohammed bin Zayed Al Nahyan and his team, and we were talking about big ideas and great ideas to help change things for children, and I presented your ideas and he wants to do it. He wants to do the whole thing."

Daniel Radek called me the next day and confirmed that indeed I had not been dreaming—Joe had been in discussion with people at the highest levels of the government. They loved the idea of the institute and wanted to structure it as a partnership between Abu Dhabi and Children's National.

The investment went from the original proposal of $100 million to $150 million. We agreed to recognize this incredible generosity by naming the institute in honor of the founding father of the United Arab Emirates,

Sheikh Zayed bin Sultan Al Nahyan. The formal announcement of the founding of the institute and our construction plan took place in September 2009. We began recruiting surgeons, doctors, and researchers in 2010.

But then, in a project filled with sudden twists and turns, we experienced another setback—our worst and most devastating one yet. During the period when we were planning the announcement, Joe began having seizures. He was diagnosed with a deadly brain tumor, a glioblastoma. Our positions suddenly changed. I became Joe's counselor now, accompanying him to appointments, explaining surgeries and treatment options, and clarifying odds. His goal, unsurprisingly, was to find a total cure for the incurable.

One time, after a round of innovative chemotherapies following brain surgery, his oncologist at the National Institutes of Health brought us images of his brain and snapped them on the box. The tumors that had been too difficult to remove in the surgery had disappeared. I could not help but say, "Holy shit."

The oncologist chuckled. "Yes, this is a holy shit moment," he said.

But this improvement in Joe's condition bought him only nine more months to live. A titan on this earth was going to fall like every man. Joe, I realized, was stunned at his fate. He was fifty-nine and felt indestructible. He said to me once, as we were leaving his oncologist's office, "I bet this damn thing began in childhood, Kurt. . . . I bet its origins lie there, in something that happened to me. Or was it in my genes? Your guys have got to figure this stuff out in kids, Kurt. You've got to get a jump on this stuff earlier."

In the months that remained to him, Joe loved to come over and check on the progress of construction and the institute. I walked down the hall once with him and the ambassador from the UAE, Yousef Al Otaiba, when Joe suddenly spotted two kids he knew from previous walk-throughs. He enjoyed stopping to chat with the patients and had grown very close to a number of them, particularly a couple of kids with cancer who were special favorites: a girl who had lost her leg to a tumor but still loved to dance, and a boy who'd had leukemia and wanted to dedicate his life to finding a cure for childhood cancer.

I couldn't help but wonder, as I watched Joe kneel to level his gaze and engage with these two patients, if the institute he had envisioned would someday prevent a child, fifty-some years on, from developing what he would soon die of.

PART III:

New Frontiers

CHAPTER 19:
Thinking Bigger

In the spring of 2011, after sixteen years as CEO of Children's National, Ned Zechman decided to retire. I heard through the grapevine that the hospital board wanted to hire a doctor or nurse as the new CEO, an emerging trend that harkened back to the early days, when children's hospitals were usually led by physicians. My work on the Joseph E. Robert, Jr., Center for Surgical Care had caught the board's attention. Several board members approached me, curious to know if I would be interested in being considered for the position of CEO.

I felt uncomfortable at first with the idea of leading the whole hospital. Medicine had become a huge business, and MBAs and consultants were in some ways better prepared than doctors to lead multimillion-dollar enterprises. But during the creation of the Sheikh Zayed Institute for Pediatric Surgical Innovation and the Joseph E. Robert, Jr., Center for Surgical Care, I had learned a great deal from Joe about strategy and leadership. I'd watched him wrestle ideas into reality and wondered if I could do the same on a hospitalwide scale. From my own work as the chief of surgery, I realized I liked to lead teams, find solutions, and think about the bigger picture. Still, I was torn: proud of what I had built but wary of stepping in over my head.

I worried that if I accepted, Joe wouldn't be happy. Nor would the man who had taught me so much of what I knew. Dr. Randolph had a distinct distaste for mixing business and medicine. He had never trusted administrators and had never wanted to be one. I felt I had to call him to discuss the proposition and suspected the reaction would not be warm.

One night after work I came home and picked up the phone before even taking off my jacket. Dr. Randolph picked up himself on only the second or third ring.

"Jud," I said, choking out his first name still, though I was now nearly sixty years old. "I have this opportunity . . ."

I knew right away that that word would raise an eyebrow, just as it had done for me years ago when Dr. Holbrook had approached me about the quality and safety project. I went on anyway, giving him the pros and cons, then stopped to hear what he would say.

"You mean you're giving up medicine?" he said.

"Well, I'm not sure . . . ," I began.

"You know as well as I that when you take a child into the OR, no administrator can come between you and that precious child," he said. "You sure you want to give that up?"

I made the case, without being completely certain that I was convinced myself.

After some soul-searching and many long discussions with Alison, I decided that seeking the job would not be a betrayal of my medical career so much as its fulfillment. Jud was right, there's nothing quite like that feeling in the OR. But I believed that in giving that up, I would be able to enhance that experience for many more surgeons and specialists and their precious children. I never received Dr. Randolph's full blessing; he never relinquished his old-school view that doctors shouldn't sell out to the business side of medicine. I'm still sensitive to the optics of spending most of my time in offices and boardrooms instead of the OR and the ER, but I've also had a chance to live up to my hunch.

Before I could go ahead and announce my candidacy, I felt I had to convince Joe that I wouldn't be abandoning the projects we had developed together. So I made one more drive out to his estate.

In his final months, Joe's favorite space had become the sunroom. It was like a greenhouse, humid and dense, with plants and trees whose leaves I had to brush aside as I made my way toward him. He sat in an oversize recliner, stacks of books and magazines within reach. He was allocating his diminishing time and energies to his family and friends. His mind stayed sharp, but his body was visibly weakening. To see a big boxer in a wheelchair was heartbreaking, but his optimism and tenacity remained.

"Joe, I think I have an opportunity to take the Sheikh Zayed Institute and your center to a new level," I began. He was all about long-term vision, and I thought my best shot at earning his blessing would be to play to that thinking.

He glanced at his mail and didn't look up.

"I was asked to throw my name in the ring for the CEO job at Children's—you probably heard Ned Zechman is retiring."

His eyes zeroed in on the page in front of him as he silently formulated his response.

In the pause, I spotted a pair of boxing gloves sitting on a bookshelf behind him and thought of a way to try again. I had just seen the mother of Miguel Gonzalez, who had been a patient of mine for nearly sixteen years, at the supermarket. From the day he was born, Miguel was known to all of us as "the fighter." I had a hunch that telling Miguel's story would be a good way of showing Joe how I could apply his lessons across the whole hospital.

"I just bumped into the mother of one of my toughest patients ever, a street brawler of a kid," I said.

Joe looked up, curious.

"You know, the great thing about my job is I get to have these long relationships with kids and families. Some operations are one and done, but the ones that really leave you thinking, the ones that change you, are the kids who need repeat procedures and monitoring over many years."

I had found my way in, and I began my tale.

The fact that Miguel was born breathing was the first miracle in his life.

Birth defects tend to snowball, and they are usually not singular and localized. When one part of an infant's anatomy develops errantly in utero, it will often trigger the abnormal development of a linked organ or system.

Miguel was born without an anus. His intestines, kidneys, and spleen were poorly developed, and his lungs were immature and barely functional. The word *congenital* is one you often hear in reference to such birth disorders. Vague in meaning and often misconstrued, the term means only that the problem was there at the moment of birth. A congenital issue is not necessarily genetic. It can result from any number of factors during pregnancy, from alcohol and nicotine use to severe stress or maternal illness.

But Miguel was also born into the arms of a woman with boundless tenacity and love. Dolores Gonzalez worked several jobs—night shifts, day shifts, and weekend shifts. English was her second language, but she had no accent whatsoever when she said the words *thank you* and *my son*.

We surgeons tend to think sequentially, planning a series of steps to address and repair a syndrome. The only way to determine the feasibility of the procedure that Miguel needed, a colostomy, was to do it. We would have to open him up to determine if we could redirect his large intestine through his abdominal wall and connect it to a "bag," which he would have to use for the rest of his life to evacuate his stool.

But the appeal of a step-by-step approach can also be misleading. In Miguel's case, each of his many ailments had its own surgical solution. The problem was the cumulative complexity of all the individual surgeries combined—and their cascading side effects. If we were successful on this first operation, he'd no longer need life support, but he would still need additional procedures to maintain life. But would this life be worth living? And who would decide?

My surgical team wanted to jump right in and start fixing things, but the neonatology team reminded us of the big picture. Its members urged us to think not just of the feasibility of the sequence of surgeries but of Miguel's overall long-term quality of life. That first morning they left a question hanging in the air: What was our goal for Miguel? What did we envision as the ultimate conclusion to years of painful and expensive medical intervention?

Later in the day, I visited Mrs. Gonzalez in the NICU. She was hovering over Miguel. The warmth radiated from his isolette, and I could see sweat on her forehead. Her kind, round face glowed in the orange light. "It is not for us to decide," she said calmly. "Don't give up on him." I was moved but unconvinced.

In a tiny room off the NICU, surgeons, neonatologists, and nurses—but not his mother—met to discuss the ethical dilemma, one that would come to the forefront more and more often as medicine continued to advance. Sitting around a table, we tried to forecast the trajectory of Miguel's life. Generally surgeons give up last—we tend to think there's a surgical solution to just about any clinical issue. I walked the team through the ten or so procedures that would be required over the next several years to push Miguel forward through life. I was confident that each operation was feasible.

The neonatologists agreed with me up to a point, but they eventually brought me around to the harsh but true reality: we could preserve Miguel's life but could not foster much quality of life. Beyond this, the costs of all of these procedures would be enormous. Miguel was covered by Medicaid, but it would reimburse to the hospital only part of the actual cost of the procedures. Children's hospitals usually make up the difference with philanthropy, to mitigate the impact on the family, but we can't do everything for everyone.

We spent the rest of the meeting talking about Miguel's mother. Working as we did in a pediatric hospital, we were accustomed to seeing uncanny devotion—feats of endurance, commitment, and insistence—from parents that could put a war hero to shame. Should we consider this mother's devotion in making our decision? Someone said, "But with a mother like that, maybe . . ." Then we let it go. We admired Mrs. Gonzalez, but at the end of the day, I think most of us saw her as an ethical complication in our recommendation. We couldn't factor love and devotion into a scientific calculus.

We decided to recommend against surgery. As we broke up the meeting and walked down the hall to tell Miguel's mother, I rehearsed my little speech, and I steeled myself to see her face full of suffering.

She stood in her customary position next to the isolette. I looked at her face and saw grace, fortitude, sadness there—and supreme tranquillity. She said nothing.

Her silence unnerved me. Without realizing it, I turned my statement into a question as it came out of my mouth. "You're sure you want to go through with this, given that it will merely be the first of many procedures? We can envision only a life for Miguel full of operations and pain. Are you sure you want to put him through that?"

I felt so tongue-tied, I was sure she thought me a fool.

"I want you to operate," she said with a strong accent. "He will make it. He will do well. Please bring me the forms."

As I watched her sign the permission and authorization forms, I told myself that at least his brain function was fine. That meant what we were about to do was ethical, if not altogether rational.

Half an hour later, as I performed the first incision, I was angry—not at Miguel's mother but at myself, for not articulating Miguel's future more clearly.

To my surprise, we discovered enough large intestine to pull through his abdomen and connect with a bag. This would be the first of many surprises that Miguel would offer up in the coming years—to everyone but his mother.

Over the next couple of years, Miguel's lungs matured and stabilized. We performed significant kidney and bowel interventions. Each time we saw Miguel, we'd notice how he was blossoming. By now he had a nurse, Linda Haga, who had become a quasi-case manager, social worker, supplemental maternal figure, and task driver all in one. Linda was the fulcrum of an increasingly effective team that was harnessing his fight and turning an impossible series of problems into an improbable, thriving life. Miguel's personality was starting to flourish along with his body: he was a big smiler, not outgoing but quick to give a high-five.

When he was ten, Miguel suffered a kidney crisis that required immediate intervention. In his preop exam, he looked at me with that serene face he had inherited from his mother and said, "Doc, just get me good enough so I can play soccer. I want to be a soccer player, and you've got to get me ready for that."

During his very first surgery I had felt anger, but this time I felt relief. We had helped a boy seize life, and his mother had helped him run with it. Now Miguel's own courage had him fantasizing about playing soccer!

After almost a decade of working with the family, Linda became a sort of second mom to him. That spring she and Mrs. Gonzalez teamed up to ask me for permission for Miguel to play soccer at a special camp for children with colostomies. At first I resisted, sometimes dodging and other times dismissing the idea. Miguel had an ostomy—a permanent bag—and I feared that one soccer ball to his belly would jeopardize years of surgical reconstruction.

But he and his mother kept badgering Linda, and Linda kept hounding me. Then in a checkup Miguel peppered me insistently in his perfect English, which his mother took such pride in. "And there is this camp for kids like me," he said. "Nurse Linda found it down in Virginia and said you can fix me so I won't get hurt. I have to play soccer, I have to play!"

His mother smiled. "Nurse Linda says you can protect the stoma," she said, her English improving, no doubt under her son's tutelage. I didn't realize that she had devised a "stoma guard" herself and sketched it out for Linda.

Finally I gave in, blessed the "stoma guard" that Linda had concocted, and held my breath the day I knew Miguel was headed off to camp.

The week went so well that he went back again the next year, and he attended soccer camp every year after that until he was too old. I imagined him, the baby for whom we'd essentially constructed a digestive system, running around like an Argentine soccer star. Dr. Randolph's old dictum—you never can tell how far a frog can jump—had no better embodiment than Miguel.

As I recounted Miguel's story to Joe, he listened intently. I went on to say that I believed the urge to rally around a child is what defines the people who choose to work at children's hospitals. Most employees, from pediatric cancer researchers to security guards, gravitate to pediatric medicine from an impulse to protect.

"I think I can take what we did together, combine that vision of a child's long life with your emphasis on innovation, and apply it not just to surgery but to research and family interaction and everything in between, Joe," I said. "Think about how much more we could do if your philosophy could transcend the entire hospital. Miguel reminds me of you. He's a fighter. Every child should be as fortunate as he was."

I told him I believed I could best honor the lessons he had taught me by building a hospital that would marry the best old-school stuff with the most exciting innovations.

"This was all your doing, Kurt," Joe said slowly when he was finally ready to speak. His tumor had slowed his speech and smile a bit, but you could still see the old fire once he locked in on his point. "You more than anyone have taught me that pediatric medicine must never forget the child while we chase the innovations that are at our fingertips." He tossed his mail on top of the magazines. "But how can I be sure that our work isn't going to lose its momentum?"

I knew that would be his main concern and told him that as CEO I would be in an even better position to drive the success of the two programs we had conceived together, because I could ensure they received the resources and leadership they needed. The work we had done together could become the blueprint for the entire hospital.

"More Miguels getting their chance to fight," he said, his eyes brightening.

"The whole place will be a big boxing ring, Joe," I said. "Every kid's team will be leaning into the ring and spurring him on."

He smiled weakly and nodded. Immediately he began to coach me for my upcoming interview. Focus on the long-term vision for each child, he said. Focus on the future of pediatric medicine. Focus on making the hospital friendlier to families. Focus on making it all comprehensible and accessible. Focus on the human touch and on the frontiers of innovation in the same sentence. Miguel shouldn't be the exception but the rule.

The following week I interviewed with the search committee and learned soon afterward that I was one of their finalists. We remaining candidates were asked to make a final pitch that would address our overarching vision for the future of the hospital and our most innovative ideas. I focused my presentation on themes that had become natural to me after so many meetings with Joe: First, create a hospital culture that enriches child and family life rather than interrupting them. Second, prioritize behavioral and mental health and the brain. And third, innovate as early in life as possible, even at the fetal stage, in order to optimize a child's adult life. These together, I decided, were the frontier of pediatric medicine.

In July 2011 the chairman of the board, Jim Lintott, called to inform me that I had been chosen. My first day on the job would be September 1, so I had a couple of months to fulfill my pledge to Joe to bolster his center and use its lessons to transform our hospital. I continued to see Joe as his health deteriorated and found myself reflecting on his own childhood and experiences growing up as a tough city kid. That summer, I tried to think of him more as a hustling and healthy boy than a dying man.

In late July and early August, I decided to visit our outposts in and around D.C. Children's National has eight specialty outpatient centers and many more primary care offices, part of a network of pediatric clinics working in underserved areas throughout the region. We also operate a number of mobile pediatric clinics, which circulate to schools and neighborhoods that don't have enough doctors or facilities to cover basic needs. Most are in Anacostia, "East of the River," where more than half of D.C.'s children live. I could hear Joe's voice in my head as I began my visits, reminding me that the hospital should be dedicated to serving *all* children in our community, particularly the ones growing up on the wrong side of the tracks or, in this case, of the river.

Driving through Anacostia, I spotted a forty-foot blue trailer with children's faces on its side and knew I had found our mobile health unit. It was parked in the middle of the Atlantic Terrace housing complex, a group of brick buildings with a sort of plaza at their center. I climbed up the bouncy steps, opened the metal door, and found Dr. Marceé White, a former resident who had impressed me a few years earlier with her energy and devotion to patients. She was examining a little boy whose throat was so red I wondered how he could even swallow.

Dr. White told me she had chosen to work here in Anacostia precisely because of little boys like this who would go for days or weeks without proper medical attention. She wanted to be where the action was and where she felt she could have the biggest impact. She said something that rings in my ears to this day:

"It's great back at the hospital, but out here on the front lines, this is where I think we can really make a difference for kids."

Dr. White's calling was to tackle the massive need for the basics—immunizations, annual physicals, and early screening for chronic diseases such as sickle cell or lead poisoning. She also wanted to help kids struggling with toxic stress and other mental health issues. Her passion caught my attention. I got the sense that she felt she was working against the current of conventional medicine, in which resources, income, and fame revolve around specialty care.

When she finished her exam, she high-fived the boy and wrote out a prescription for long-overdue antibiotics. He had strep throat, something that would have likely been recognized and treated in the other Washington, west of the Anacostia, within twenty-four hours, but here it had gone untreated for five days.

Sensing my interest, Dr. White invited me to visit the headquarters of our mobile health program, located in a creative development called THEARC. It is located in ward 8, east of the Anacostia River. The developers, Chris Smith and his partner, Skip McMahon, who founded the nonprofit Building Bridges Across the River, decided to bring together in one location a number of nonprofits—the Washington Ballet, the Levine School of Music, the Boys and Girls Clubs, a charter school, as well as a primary care clinic run by Children's National. Dr. White introduced me to her team. It was made up not just of doctors and nurses but also of social workers, parent navigators, family services associates, and psychologists—all devoted to caring for the whole child.

Before stopping to speak to the kids and their parents, she took me by the elbow and said, "Let's go for a ride."

We jumped into a dental van, which I soon learned provided oral health services throughout the community. Dental disease is the most common infectious condition in children, particularly among kids who grow up poor. Many end up with severe tooth and gum disease, which can have long-term effects on their overall health by triggering inflammation and chronic infections. Dental services are either not covered or poorly reimbursed by public insurance programs such as Medicaid, and there are few dentists across the river.

As Dr. White spoke to the driver I realized he was the famous Mr. Larry, renowned at the hospital for his grandfatherly attentiveness to patients and staff alike and for his good deeds, gently redirecting troubled youth and putting in countless hours of overtime during flu season. At one point on our tour of the neighborhood, Dr. White signaled for him to stop. He slammed on the brakes and as the van heaved, I got the sense this was a regular occurrence. Dr. White pointed at a mother pushing a child in a stroller with a couple of toddlers straggling behind her.

"Let me cut them off," Mr. Larry said, pulling forward and stopping the van in the middle of an intersection.

Dr. White jumped out and gave the mother a hug. Their conversation got animated after that. I could tell she was really giving her a talking to.

"She's angry?" I half stated and half asked Mr. Larry.

"You bet she is," he said with a belly laugh. "Dr. White don't like it when kids miss an appointment. And when they miss a bunch of them—oh, boy."

"It looked like you gave that mother a bit of a tongue-lashing," I said, when she finally returned. Dr. White laughed and shook her head. She told me she had cared for the mother as a teenager and was now the pediatrician for her children. She didn't like the fact that her kids had missed their last few appointments.

"And what did she say?" I asked.

"Tomorrow at nine o'clock," Dr. White said matter-of-factly. "Larry, I heard it might go up to one hundred tomorrow, so you may have to pick them up."

Mr. Larry nodded with a smile. I was beginning to think that Dr. White was a newfangled version of Dr. Ong, a devoted community doctor.

Driving home that night, I thought about Joe Robert, but also about those dedicated ladies back in 1870 who had founded Children's Hospital to take care of orphaned and crippled children. What would they have made of the vast network their creation had become? I had been thinking a lot since being named CEO about what it takes to be a top children's hospital. As with colleges and universities, the most influential ranking of hospitals is offered by *U.S. News & World Report.* Their main criteria are outcomes and volume of cases for each specialty, and what is called "reputation." But there is no ranking for delivering primary care to the community. How were Dr. White and her team—and similar teams across the country—valued and scored? How did caring for the whole community and addressing issues such as infant mortality, mental health, and preventive care factor into the evaluation of a hospital's excellence?

Not long after my visit to Anacostia, Children's National participated in a community health needs assessment that included most of Washington's hospitals and many families and community organizations. We asked people what they felt they needed most from their hospitals. I was taken aback, after so many years in surgery, with their answers. They had nothing to do with excellence in specialty care or cutting-edge treatment. Parents prioritized mental health services, health literacy, the coordination of care for chronic diseases, and problems such as diabetes, obesity, and asthma, which were plaguing the community.

As I pondered the results, visions of the children bustling in and out of

Dr. White's mobile health unit kept popping into my head. These kids were getting checkups and screenings and immunizations—the sorts of things parents were begging for more of.

The big idea that grew out of this survey and my visits to Anacostia was to reorganize the hospital. When I started in my new position in the fall, I decided to restructure hospital leadership and elevate the head of primary care, Dr. Denice Cora-Bramble, to chief medical officer. This may seem like a simple shift, but it was really a radical signal that specialty care and primary care would receive the same focus and resources. Dr. Cora-Bramble's innovations would ensure that serving every child in our community, not just the ones suffering from rare conditions, would be our priority, regardless of how it affected our national ranking and reputation. We'd make curing strep throat and screening for lead or toxic stress as passionate a focus as cancer research and minimally invasive surgery.

I kept Joe apprised of these changes even as his health steadily declined. His delight at each update inspired me to double down on our new direction. He loved the nitty-gritty of pediatric care as much as the high-flying research and innovations, and knew enough about the hospital by now to appreciate that their symbolic union at the top of our leadership structure would mean real transformation.

One night in early December, Joe's family called me. He was under home hospice care and was fading fast. I made a final trip to see him. I held his hand for a while and whispered to him that I would do my best to help everyone around me fulfill his vision. I didn't tell him how much I would miss him. I didn't tell him how much I had learned from him. I simply told him his vision would endure. He died that night, and my real work began the next day.

CHAPTER 20:
Navigating the Hospital

One day that August before I had become CEO, I went to a neighborhood barbecue at a park near our house. A few friends had heard the news of my appointment, and they came up to congratulate me. While I stood talking with them, another friend, Beverly, made a beeline toward me. Her teenage son Benjamin had very severe autism, and he regularly came to Children's National for medical care.

"Kurt, I'm pissed and I'm hurt," Beverly said, tears welling up in her eyes. I peered at my friends and could feel I was blushing. "Our family refuses ever to go back to your hospital. I don't want this to affect our friendship, but you need to know our experience was dreadful! I am afraid Ben is going to suffer long-term consequences."

I bit my tongue as I tried to remember if I had managed any aspect of her son's care recently. My neighbors gave us a little space to talk. Beverly collected herself, and I apologized and urged her to tell me what had happened.

Benjamin had come in for two procedures, one to his fix ingrown toenails and the other a teeth cleaning. His autism was so severe he required anesthesia for both—he had a violent reaction to being touched by strangers. Successfully orchestrating even a single procedure under anesthesia for a child with severe autism is difficult, but coordinating two, one involving a dentist and the other a surgeon, can generate huge stress for both the family and the child. Beverly had made multiple calls to the hospital's different clinics to align the schedule so the two procedures could be done simultaneously, but unable to overcome the bureaucracy, she had given up. Benjamin was subjected to two trips to the hospital and two separate sedations.

"It would be easier and more efficient, not to mention cheaper for all of you, to coordinate these appointments more humanely," Beverly said. "Just think of the toll it takes on your nurses to get Ben ready to be put to sleep on two separate occasions for such simple procedures. Can you imagine how he reacted the second time around? And how do you think I felt, seeing him suffer and rage like that?"

Her anger was surging again. But instead of focusing on Beverly and her son, all I could think was that there must be thousands of mothers in the United States in her same situation. I was hearing this only because we lived in the same neighborhood. What about the families who didn't bump into their doctors over hot dogs and watermelon?

"I'll look into it," I said, falling back on the cliché that so often popped out of my mouth in moments of embarrassment. But then I remembered Dr. Randolph's warning that I should *own it* and added, "In the end, I am responsible."

As surgeon in chief, I had been in a position to address her son's situation because I managed the surgical specialists as well as the anesthesiologists and the operating rooms. I thought I had been a pretty good surgeon in chief, but I hadn't focused on the unique mechanics of scheduling for autism spectrum children and hadn't really looked into how well the surgery department was coordinating with other departments. I quickly realized that Beverly was giving me my first big lesson in what I would face as CEO. In recent years, dozens of family friends had come to me with stories of behavioral and psychological issues in their children. I had made mental health a key part of my presentation to the search committee, and now I would have to walk the talk.

With the help of several nursing colleagues, I began to think through what it might take to help Beverly and her son, and so many others like them. Obviously we would have to create a new position, but what exactly would it require?

The person would need a deep knowledge of the clinics—each specialty, ranging from dermatology to cardiology, has outpatient spaces and offices where doctors evaluate children and meet parents—and of the hospital building's complex operation and layout. That was a tall order. Medicine is so specialized that we rarely look up from the field we're plowing. Another requirement for the job was a keen sensitivity to the psychological and emotional needs of children and their families, particularly kids suffering from autism spectrum disorders or other mental health problems. The person would need great coordination skills and be able to identify bureaucratic roadblocks and foresee conflicts among providers.

One night not long after my encounter with Beverly, I was having dinner with Alison at home and we were lamenting the news that a close friend had been diagnosed with an aggressive breast cancer. We counted all the friends we had heard from lately who had been diagnosed with breast cancer. We talked about how the dozen or so of them had all been overwhelmed as much by negotiating medical care as by the treatment itself. At a time of immense stress, every one of them had struggled to figure out how to get the best care and whether to choose radiation therapy, chemotherapy, and/or surgery.

Historically, few resources were available to guide them to the right decision, but some cancer hospitals had started to employ a new class of nurses called nurse navigators to help breast cancer patients negotiate their complex treatment pathways. Several friends told us how grateful they had been to have had this resource. Suddenly it clicked—that was exactly what we needed at Children's!

"My nurse navigator saved my life as much as the radiation and chemo," one friend had told Alison. "She is the reason I am cancer free. Without her, I would have made the wrong choices and gotten sicker from all the stress of making appointments and coordinating blood work and exams."

I lay awake that night, convinced I'd had my first significant vision for the treatment of mental and behavioral health. The next morning I asked my team to do an in-depth study of the role of nurse navigators at cancer centers. I had a hunch we could apply the concept to help families with children on the autism spectrum—and other patients with complex diseases or special coordination needs.

The problem was, insurance companies would never offset the cost of such a position. We would surely improve clinical outcomes and decrease expenses, but we would never be able to justify the nurse navigator's salary with a line item or a reimbursement code. We knew, even before we identified who would fill the position, that the job would require philanthropic support to sustain it.

Working with our philanthropy team, we received some pilot funding from two of our most generous supporters, Betty and Chuck Ewing. They immediately grasped the benefits of this concept and pledged to help us develop the position and strategy. My nursing colleagues and I wrote a job description and titled the position "pediatric nurse navigator." I knew the position's success at breast cancer centers would resonate strongly.

Then we set about trying to identify a person with the right combination of experience and charisma to interact with medical professionals, coax them, and occasionally boss them around on behalf of families—and enough courage to sensitively but firmly deal with parents who aren't always ready to accept that there are limits to what we can do. The person would have to be like a head coach, overseeing a bunch of assistant coaches and star players in a moving choreography of schedules, needs, talents, egos, and ambitions, all in the service of making a child and his or her family's life easier.

It wasn't long before I zeroed in on Eileen Walters. Eileen was a hematology-oncology nurse who had always bonded well with patients. They seemed to want her in the room whenever I had to do anything that was painful. Eileen worked only night shifts, so our encounters were pretty infrequent. She had five children of her own, which explained her choice of schedule. She wanted to be there in the mornings when they woke up and in the afternoons when they came home from school.

That spring, as part of a fund-raiser called Be Brave and Shave, I lined up on a stage in the hospital atrium alongside board members, other docs, a few nurses, and a handful of patients. We had all collected pledges that would go to our cancer program if we shaved our heads. The haircutters were ready for us. A photographer snapped photos as strands of hair fell to the floor. Later that week someone posted the photos to the hospital Web site. The next day Eileen sent me an email, teasing me about shaving my already bald head. She had the perfect mix of skills, and I encouraged her to apply for the job.

"Until you told me, I didn't know that this position had never been applied to specialty pediatric care," Eileen told me later. "So I took some time to study the origins of nurse navigators, their effectiveness in streamlining breast cancer care and raising its quality and effectiveness. Once I understood, I could imagine the possibilities for children and their families, and I knew I wanted the job."

She started her new job soon after I started mine, and our joint focus on helping families navigate the hospital became my first significant initiative as CEO. Children needing mental and behavioral care naturally became the predominant focus, so I was pleased to be fulfilling the commitment I had made to the board.

Eileen's first case was a toddler named Stephen, who was autistic and had a terminal genetic condition that slowed his body's ability to process fats. He was also suffering from a form of PTSD as a result of the many interventions we'd had to perform. This time he needed surgery for a kidney issue, but multiple specialists were involved with his care, including Dr. Tony Sandler, who had replaced me as surgeon in chief. Stephen's mother wanted to be sure that everyone on his extensive medical team knew he was having surgery, and she wanted the whole team's specialized recommendations for the surgery and recovery.

Eileen communicated with all the specialists involved in Stephen's care and set up evaluations to ensure that the surgery and recovery protocols would take into account the safety precautions called for by his rare genetic condition. Following the surgery, she coordinated Stephen's ongoing care. During his stay, she taught his mother how to organize his medical information, explained what additional support services were available at the hospital, and created a contact list to coordinate Stephen's appointments.

I met Stephen's mother one day at an autism conference being held at the hospital. She walked intently toward me, and for a moment I had the same sensation I'd had that day at the picnic when Beverly darted in my direction. "My life is immensely easier because of this nurse navigator," she said. "But what makes me happiest is the decrease in my son's stress. I believe he senses that I'm less stressed, and that makes him relax, too."

Not long after helping Stephen, Eileen worked with Beverly's son Benjamin. A few months later I saw Beverly on a morning walk, and she again made a beeline toward me—this time with a big smile on her face.

"Gosh, how things have improved with this nurse navigator thing, Kurt," she said. "You can see I'm happier, but you should see Ben."

It was the first compliment I'd received from a friend in my tenure as CEO. As I walked home, I thought of Dr. Randolph's advice the first time I'd had to operate on a friend's child—"You're the best guy for the job," he'd said—precisely because I was their friend. The concept of teamwork and the idea of involving parents as team members—lessons I learned early in my career—form the foundation of the nurse navigator position. Eileen readily admits that she is only as good as the parent who decides to take advantage of her services.

Many children's hospitals are now embracing the prototype of the nurse navigator, making thousands of people's lives easier in a way that only pediatric specialty centers can. The navigator helps parents identify and manage the child's team and ensures that they have full awareness of and access to the hospital's resources. Rather than increase costs, the position ultimately makes treatments more efficient and cost effective—yet her work still isn't covered by insurance. For me, the navigator role is a symbol of a radical rethinking we should invest in as a society for the health of our children. Nurse navigators are more than worthwhile using any sort of calculus—treatment results, emotional well-being, or financial accounting.

I had found success with one program, but Joe's voice was silently egging me on to make a bigger, hospitalwide transformation.

CHAPTER 21:
Mental Health

Being a community doctor means being perpetually on call—and not just at the hospital. Taking calls from friends and neighbors at all hours—for everything from a splinter to a severe allergic reaction—was one of the most gratifying parts of my job, and once I became CEO I urged people to keep calling me—not least because if they didn't, I would miss it so much. My concern proved to be unfounded: the calls for advice kept coming, and each one reminded me that a doctor plays a special function in a community, like a good rabbi or priest. For many of us in pediatrics, this sense of service, of ministering to families in need, makes up for our lower salaries. The degree to which most pediatricians I know embrace this role distinguishes pediatric care as a field apart, a calling as much as a profession.

A month or so into my tenure as CEO, at around eleven p.m. on a Friday night, the phone rang. Our sons were both out, so Alison and I glanced at each other as parents of teenage children do. I picked up and found my friend Tom Johnson, the father of a smart and attractive fourteen-year-old girl who socialized with my younger son, was on the line. We were buddies and played in a softball league together, and I had always enjoyed his easygoing manner. My heart beat faster.

But Tom's call had nothing to do with our son. His daughter Catherine was lying in bed in a stupor, and he had no idea what to do. They had been to her pediatrician that afternoon, and Catherine had been diagnosed with anorexia. As Tom told me the specifics, I realized he didn't fully understand the gravity of the situation. I asked him to take his daughter's pulse rate and the results frightened me. I was worried Catherine was in a life-threatening situation. Her heart rate was in the fifties, and her father could barely feel her pulse. She needed to be hospitalized immediately.

I had seen Tom regularly, and there had never been any indication that his daughter was having problems. On the contrary, I'd heard she was doing extremely well in school, was thriving in athletics, and was getting ready to look at colleges.

But I shouldn't really have been shocked. Over the last few years I had received more and more calls related to mental health issues. People didn't seem to know what to do or how to find good help. Nationally there weren't enough psychiatrists and psychologists, or outpatient clinics and long-term support systems, to handle the huge uptick in behavioral and mental health problems. What's more, many hospitals had been closing their inpatient units, so the physical resources were diminishing too, just as the number of patients was multiplying.

The unifying theme across most of these cases was that the families had been in denial. There is still such a stigma around mental health that often parents won't recognize a problem or admit it exists until it reaches a state of crisis, and that seemed to be what had happened with Tom. Catherine's pediatrician had previously told him and his wife that she needed to be hospitalized, but they hadn't heeded her urging.

I couldn't understand why the pediatrician hadn't made arrangements herself rather than leave it up to the family. Anorexia nervosa, the technical term for the eating disorder, has a mortality rate that ranges from 5 percent in children and adolescents to 20 percent in older patients, so the stakes were high. On the phone I reassured Tom that in my experience, most anorexia emergencies could be resolved over time through therapy with the commitment of the entire family. But we had to get Catherine into a hospital, where we could address the life-threatening dimension of the problem with fluids and nutrition.

I hung up and called over to the hospital, my heart aching for Tom. Eating disorders are often manifestations of deeper issues, like depression or anxiety, and I imagined the long and difficult journey Tom and his wife were about to embark on with their daughter.

When I called our inpatient psychiatric unit, I was barraged with questions about the family's insurance plan and was asked for the pediatrician's paperwork. And I was the CEO! I could only imagine what most parents would go through. Apparently resources were at such a premium that our unit was stretched to the limit, and many insurance companies didn't cover psychiatric care or had major limitations on their coverage. The admissions team needed to understand the parameters of Catherine's insurance coverage before they could admit her. There was no question that they would take her, but admitting her without the proper paperwork because it was late at night and the case was urgent would never cut it once the reimbursement conversation started.

After a couple of awkward calls back and forth with Tom, the admissions team decided that because this was a life-threatening situation, they would take the case regardless of whether the insurance would cover it. They would fight it out on behalf of the family to press the insurance company to provide the necessary coverage. This sort of situation has become an unpleasant fact of life for families of patients suffering from behavioral and mental health conditions and for us at the hospital. There is just no good health policy around coverage.

I called ahead to the emergency department, so they were ready to receive Catherine and her family. Then I went back to bed, satisfied that I'd been able to help a friend. But I couldn't get back to sleep. I lay in bed thinking about what Tom and Catherine must be going through and wondering how so many families could be left to shoulder the burden on their own.

Over 20 percent of children will have a mental health issue at some point in their lives, and eight years on average pass from the time the first symptoms are noticed to the time treatment begins. We are failing as a society to prioritize early recognition and diagnosis—both of which make mental health issues much easier to correct.

As part of my interview for the CEO job, I had pitched this big idea of a mind/brain institute, which would focus on getting children with mental issues and their families the care they needed on par with care for more tangible physical ailments and conditions. I envisioned a new campus where neurological research would be integrated with clinical care. I hoped the institute could take a leading role in advocating for new policies around children's mental health.

About a year after I became CEO and six months after Tom's call, the school shooting in Sandy Hook, Connecticut, took place, galvanizing this effort for me. The massacre threw into stark relief the fact that children and their families were not getting the care they needed soon enough to prevent tragedy. I was so upset that I wrote an op-ed in the *Washington Post* pleading for more funding for mental health research and behavioral care. At the same time, I worked with my team to plan a pediatric mental health summit. We envisioned using our bully pulpit in the nation's capital to bring together the leaders of children's hospitals and child psychiatry units nationwide.

Catherine's case was a potent reminder that for all our big ideas, every day there are children in crisis who need our help. The day after she was admitted, I had to travel to a conference in Chicago and didn't hear anything from Tom over the next few days. I am always hesitant to intrude on parents' privacy if they don't talk to me.

The day I returned to the office, Tom showed up. I saw him talking to the receptionist, clearly very upset. His face was red, and his manner animated. When he saw me, instead of his usual friendly greeting, he gave me an accusatory look. I invited him into my office, and even before we sat down, he was challenging me.

"Kurt, I'm so disappointed in this hospital." He looked me straight in the eye. "Have you been to the inpatient psychiatric unit? Well, I hope you haven't, because if you had, you would've done something about it. It's just not right for kids with behavioral issues. They need the same type of facilities that kids with physical diseases have. It's just not right. You need to do something about it."

Several years earlier we had built a new inpatient tower (the Joseph E. Robert, Jr., Center was the surgical component) to take care of patients with medical and surgical diseases. But the psychiatry unit had not been included in the plan and was still in the same location—it had not even been renovated. The rooms were not private. The facilities for group therapy were dark and windowless. The amenities for parents were sparse.

I felt profoundly embarrassed. Here I had been advocating for a transformation for pediatric mental and behavioral health, but my own hospital was falling short. These patients and their families felt shortchanged. We weren't practicing what we were preaching. I had a great stump speech about a glorious concept of mental health care, but the work I needed to do right here at home was real—and hard.

I vowed to Tom that we would transform our facilities.

I had previously managed to lure Kathy Gorman, my partner in the quality data analysis work (see Chapter 16), back as our new chief operating officer. She was the first person I called. Kathy, her team, and I went on to develop a plan to raise money to build a new unit or a new campus for the Mind/Brain Institute and to recruit psychologists, psychiatrists, and neurologists to do research. But we just could not get traction. We had some small wins over a couple of years, and a few donors generously stepped forward to help renovate the activity room used for inpatients. We had already created an endowed chair for the psychiatry department, but we just couldn't generate the kind of snowballing philanthropic interest that we needed to renovate and enhance the whole facility and create the Mind/Brain Institute.

Then one day about three years later, I bumped into Tom and Catherine at an electronics store near my house. They were laughing together, and

Catherine looked up at me and smiled. I felt relieved. Tom shook my hand, his callouses betraying a life in construction work. He had formed his own company right out of high school and now ran one of the most successful residential building firms in the area. I wanted to ask Catherine how she was feeling but held to my rule to let the parent or patient initiate the conversation.

"Look at my girl—how healthy she is, eh, doc?" Tom said. They beamed at each other, and Catherine told me she was getting ready to do a semester abroad in Sweden.

"How are you guys doing over there, Kurt?" Tom asked. "I'm tempted to bring my drills and saws and renovate that psychiatric unit with my own crew one of these days."

Then it dawned on me. Tom had a bit of Joe Robert's tough-guy garrulousness in him, and he was a native Washingtonian to boot. Maybe he was the man to get the job done.

"Let's have a beer sometime soon, Tom," I said. "I need to talk with you."

Soon thereafter we met at a local pub, and Tom gave me the details of his daughter's courageous recovery. They had undergone extensive family therapy, working with a psychologist who helped them talk more openly about Catherine's issues. She attended peer group therapy with other young women who came together to discuss their hopes and fears. A psychiatrist at Children's National managed her medication for depression over a two-year period, then slowly weaned her off it. She, and they, had dedicated their lives to fixing hers.

Tom offered me a detailed account of the strengths and weaknesses of our psychiatric unit, and he agreed to spearhead a philanthropic campaign to raise the funds for a full-scale renovation. He didn't have Joe Robert's deep pockets, but he was an even stronger arm-twister, and over the course of six months we were able to raise a significant portion of the required funding. Tom reminded me that a children's hospital belongs to the community, depends on its members, and needs them as much as they need it.

That summer we organized the Pediatric Mental Health Summit and brought together the leaders of a number of children's hospitals with pediatric mental health experts. These two entities—hospitals and the psychiatric community—had existed in relatively separate universes. The hospital leaders recognized that they needed to engage their pediatric psychiatry divisions with more energy and clarity, and those working in mental health emerged knowing that they had to lobby more aggressively for themselves. The event was a huge success, and its goal of increasing communication resonated on both sides.

We followed up with a second summit two years later, and that one contributed to legislation that increased funding for pediatric mental health and created better access and awareness.

Meanwhile, at Children's National, we began placing psychologists and psychiatrists in the same outpatient clinics as our primary care doctors, so that when one of our general pediatricians identified a psychiatric problem, the child could be seen right away. We also began a pilot project using telemedicine, so that pediatricians could get immediate access to a child psychiatrist or psychologist through a teleconsultation. These are all baby steps, but the tide is slowly turning, and I remain hopeful that the big idea of the Mind/Brain Institute can be fulfilled.

I had started out by attacking the big picture, then was forced to focus on needs and deficiencies closer to home. Now that our own house was more in order, it was time to take the next step. As a hospital, we would have to help solve the larger national crisis in pediatric mental health care. The signs of trouble are everywhere—suicides, violence, anxiety disorders, eating disorders, and attention deficit problems. Mental health issues are some of the largest and least soluble of all problems in pediatrics, but they are now so prevalent that we must tackle them with the same seriousness and determination with which we tackle complex diseases like cancer.

Mental health is one of the last great frontiers in medicine, but we are not approaching it with enough moxie or resources. So many problems remain with insurance coverage and the training of mental health providers that I and my colleagues at pediatric hospitals across the nation find ourselves at a standstill. Scattershot fund-raising and philanthropy can take us only so far. Maybe parents like Tom, shaped and organized into an army of concerned families nationwide, will be able to trigger the political and cultural change that will be necessary to save our kids and transform our society.

CHAPTER 22:
A Child's Life

I knew right away when Nathan stood up to speak that Kathy Gorman had set me up.

In 2009 Kathy had left Children's National to become chief of nursing at the Children's Hospital of Philadelphia. When I became CEO, I persuaded her to come back to be my chief operating officer (COO). The COO makes a hospital run, overseeing everything from facilities management to relationships with insurance companies. I loved the idea of a doctor and a nurse having the two top jobs at Children's National, both for the message it sent parents and the staff and for the insider knowledge it would bring when it came time to innovate.

Kathy accepted, and one of her first moves as COO was to hold town hall meetings with patients and their families in our auditorium. She invited me to an early one, and it started off well. The seats filled up, and parents and kids were smiling and energetic. Kathy seemed to have found a way to build a sense of community in a place that is transitory by nature.

But public events like this can go awry, as I realized when Nathan stood up, adjusted his IV, and began to speak. "Look at these paint colors and balloons," he began. "The little kids love them. The problem is, a lot of us here aren't little kids. We're teenagers. I love my nurses and doctors, but to tell you the truth, I'm bored stiff."

I shifted in my chair, glanced at Kathy, and received a slight, knowing smile in return. I turned back to Nathan, who was unquestionably addressing me directly.

"You've done nothing to really make the lives of teenagers easier," he continued. "When I was a patient in Philadelphia, they had this music studio we all loved. They had games for us and activities. We've outgrown *Sesame Street*, you know."

Kathy stood to engage him—I suppose she had seen me suffer enough. But the point was taken, and afterward I approached Nathan and asked him about adolescent programs at Children's Hospital of Philadelphia (CHOP). The music studio, I learned, was called Seacrest Studios, and Ryan Seacrest, host of *American Idol*, was supporting the rollout of such studios at several children's hospitals nationwide.

I met with Kathy afterward and challenged her to bring Seacrest Studios to Children's National. As soon as I'd done so, I realized this had been a trap. Kathy had been the chief of nursing at CHOP for three years before I hired her away. She had obviously wanted me to hear from a child rather than from her how transformative the studio could be.

"By the way, I love these town halls," I told Kathy. "Keep them coming."

I had used a number of arguments in my effort to persuade Kathy to serve as my COO. The town hall had brought one of them to life right before my eyes: a person can do more for kids and their families when running the whole hospital and not just the nursing department. Kathy had proven to be a tough audience. She loved the front lines of nursing as much as I loved surgery, and she kept coming back to how her gig in Philly allowed her to put the nurse-family relationship at the forefront. But in the end she relented.

She spent her first months on the job canvassing nurses for advice and heard a surprising pattern: make our Child Life program more of a priority. The Child Life team manages children's activities. In essence, it is a mental health provider, for sick and hospitalized children need diversions and fun to maintain their well-being and optimize their healing. Our specialists were dedicated and productive, but the nurses wanted to see their work better integrated into the overall medical team. Kathy and I decided this would require two key steps: linking the Child Life department with the nursing, surgical, facilities, and all other departments, and making technology and social media a fundamental part of the whole child and family experience. Kathy's goal was to make our hospital as well known for its Child Life program as for its surgery and radiology departments. And that fit right in with the Mind/Brain Institute idea and my new focus on mental health.

Given medicine's hierarchies and snobberies, making Child Life such a priority was more controversial than it might seem. Frequently in hospitals, doctors look down their noses at "non-MDs." We surgeons are definitely the most arrogant, and the pecking order runs downhill from us. For some, a master's degree in social work can trigger eye-rolling.

But Kathy cut through this superficial nonsense. In addition to balancing the books and explaining our costs to insurance companies, she had to ensure that Children's National fostered a culture that embraced the joy and wonder of childhood and the value of play. These are two key objectives of Child Life precisely because they are so essential to a happy child's life.

It still stuns me how few parents who come to our hospital even know Child Life exists. As parents, we study our kids' schools, rec leagues, and teachers, but we put little time into understanding what health care they will receive and how to manage it for optimal success. Who will your child's doctor or surgeon be if they have an accident or need urgent care? How can you be confident that they are good? What will the nursing schedule look like? Thanks to Kathy, parents can now visit the hospital, meet with Child Life specialists, and even take a tour—with their child, if they want—to eliminate a lot of anxiety.

Child Life specialists take the language of medicine and translate it into words that kids can understand so they feel less afraid. When I was a surgeon, it took me years to realize that the slightest word or gesture could send a child off into a land of dangerous and excessive imagination. A Child Life specialist helps the entire team understand that kids' active imaginations cause unnecessary distress if we don't speak to them in their own words.

When you tell a five-year-old she is going to have a CAT scan, do you know what she is most likely to think about? Cats. Kids interpret what they hear as they understand the world. Not long ago we had a young girl who required abdominal surgery. The doctors discussed the surgery at her bedside with her parents as the girl listened attentively. After the doctors left, she screamed whenever anyone in a white coat entered her room, and she refused to eat. The Child Life specialist discovered, by playing a gardening game with her, that she thought she had a seed in her stomach that the doctors wanted to remove, and she had convinced herself that if she didn't eat, it wouldn't grow. The doctor had tried to downplay the significance of the surgery by joking that they had to remove a seed from her belly or else it was going to grow into a flower. She had taken his joke literally. The Child Life specialist was able to reassure her once the mystery was solved.

In her first two years as COO, Kathy prioritized building up the Child Life program but also worked on bringing in Seacrest Studios. Several local supporters gave us significant philanthropic support—enough to supplement Ryan Seacrest's contributions—and construction in the main atrium was completed in 2015. The programming at the studio is almost exclusively child generated and is broadcast daily to every room from ten a.m. to four p.m. It starts with the *Brooks and Morgan Morning Show* (a variety show where kids can perform) and also includes regular programs like *Hospital Bingo, Craft Tuesday,* and *Hunter's Sports Wrap Up*. (Hunter, a discharged patient who comes back to host his show, recently interviewed Olympic swimmer Katie Ledecky on it.)

Seacrest Studios was crucial for the healing of a fourteen-year-old girl named Ellie. She had been diagnosed with Crohn's disease, an inflammatory bowel disease that causes severe discomfort and that is increasing in frequency for unknown reasons. In a child, complications from Crohn's are sometimes more pronounced than in adults and often require surgery. The disease disrupted Ellie's sleep and her diet, and she was suffering from severe weight loss and exhaustion.

We checked Ellie into the hospital to help her gain back weight—she was hovering on the edge of the danger zone. But gaining weight is not as simple as inserting a couple of IVs. Striking the right balance between medication and nutrition is difficult, involving trial and error, and it can lead to some horrendous nights. Sometimes it can take months to get the balance right, and that was what happened with Ellie. Medicines and nutrients were flowing into her through two IVs and a PICC (peripherally inserted central catheter) line, a special IV for long-term intravenous access. She had to carry an IV backpack whenever she left her room so her nutrition infusion would not be interrupted. After a couple of weeks of this regimen, she was sleeping only a few hours each night because of the uncontrollable, violent vomiting it caused, and she was starting to lose her spirit.

Brooks Looney, a Child Life specialist who works extensively in the Seacrest Studios, was assigned to help Ellie. She worked with her nurses to get her into a wheelchair so that she could come down to the studio. The change in Ellie was almost immediate. For the first time in weeks, she smiled. Her rigid body relaxed a bit. At last she was being distracted from her sickness.

"The studio connects with all the patients' rooms, and we run music shows and skits and even Trivial Pursuit–type games that allow everyone to participate," Brooks told me. "And while the show was airing, we taught Ellie how to use some of the equipment on the recording side of the studio. Then a few days later, we let her work with a deejay. It wasn't so much the music or the technology that hooked her as the vibe of the place, the people and the activities and the friends she started to make. It was so thrilling to see her take her mind off her pain."

As Ellie's doctors and nurses scheduled her treatments and procedures, Brooks told them that these studio visits would have to take priority. So her medical team built her treatment schedule around the schedule of the

Seacrest Studios. When I saw Ellie giggling in front of a microphone in the studio one day, I felt Joe Robert was giving us a double thumbs-up from above.

One day Ellie's mom called Brooks and me aside in the studio. "I don't think you understand what you're doing here," her mom said. "She was up sick all night, she slept for about two hours, but at nine a.m. she was ready for her morning shower so she could get down here. She's even planning a radio show with her friend down the hall."

We're looking forward to Ellie's creative contribution. While her doctors are confident they will find the right balance of medicine and nutrition to check her Crohn's disease yet allow her to live a more normal life, we've found that bringing in a little bit of normalcy from the outside is actually helping expedite her treatments.

Those of us working on the front lines of pediatric care know these programs can help children heal faster. But how can we convince insurance providers of their financial logic? Child Life is increasingly a priority at children's hospitals all over the country, and many of my fellow pediatric leaders are now making this case. Ellie and countless other patients have shaped our Child Life program and helped transform medicine from an experience with a tunnel focus on health care into a team sport committed to preserving all dimensions of childhood during medical treatment.

After we worked to improve our mental health and Child Life focus, our building blocks were in place and we were ready for more. I felt that innovations were necessary in the old-school world of human interaction as much as at the forefront of medical investigation. It may not sound cutting-edge to say so, but the two go hand in hand. I was convinced that the brave new frontier of pediatric care combined Dr. Randolph's folksy lessons with Joe Robert's bold visions. Innovation on both fronts would be equally essential.

CHAPTER 23:
What You Don't Know

Almost every time I walk through our NICU I hear stories that follow the same disconcerting arc: parents should have identified a high-quality NICU before birth and now find their baby being transferred to us because of complications at another facility. With a new, fragile life, time is of the essence, and these parents' lack of knowledge often leads to hairy situations. So why don't parents know more?

A few years ago, a longtime friend from my book club sent me a text message at about nine a.m. one summer weekday. I was getting ready for a tough meeting with members of the board about our annual budget, when a photo pinged on my phone: Greg's blue-eyed and big-footed newborn twins. It gave me a real boost. Greg and Alicia had been struggling to conceive, and like many older parents whose fertility doctors implant multiple fertilized eggs, they now found themselves with twins. Both had been through tragic losses of immediate family members, which made this expansion of their family all the more meaningful. Greg was haunted by his brother's death at a young age; he had told me that the arrival of twin boys promised to make up for this loss.

"A solid six pounds each," the text message read. The doctor in me gave the boys, Ezekiel and Lukas, a good eyeing up and down. They looked healthy and alert, and I went to show my longtime assistant, Carol Manning, the picture. Carol, knowing full well that multiple births can be associated with complications, asked where they had been born and I named a hospital in Maryland with a pretty strong NICU. Greg told me they had chosen the hospital after hearing the dreadful term "high risk" that medicine applies to all twin pregnancies. They might need a specialized center for the boys' first few days, he reasoned, despite positive results from Alicia's regular sonograms and the fact that she had carried the boys without complications for thirty-eight weeks.

Like most new parents, Greg and Alicia had no plan in case of unforeseen complications. I should have given them my standard spiel about how every parent-to-be needs to have an emergency plan in place, study their insurance coverage to determine which children's hospital is covered in case something goes wrong, specify the location of the hospital, and have their transport there mapped out. But I didn't want to seem pushy and had let it go.

NICUs are ranked by the American Academy of Pediatrics according to the resources they can provide (from Level I to IV, with Level IV NICUs offering the most extensive care). Greg and Alicia had selected a NICU with a solid Level III ranking. Level IIIs do well with standard cases of prematurity, but Level IVs are best for crises that require pediatric surgical specialists and more sophisticated technology. They did not research where the nearest Level IV was located or discuss with their obstetrician what might trigger the need for a transfer to a Level IV. Nor had they confirmed with their hospital whether there was a 24/7 communication system in place with a Level IV. No parent wants to hear it, but numerous crises can emerge during a baby's first hours and days—even when Apgar scores and initial exams suggest all is well.

During the pregnancy, Greg had told Carol, who is from Jamaica, that he played lots of Bob Marley and the Wailers for the boys in utero. When she saw the photo, Carol told me it was fitting that they both seemed to be wailing.

I went through my day, wondering every now and then about the twins, but in my line of work no news is generally good news, and I took comfort in the fact that I hadn't heard from Greg. I drove home that night and showed the photo to Alison, who looked the boys up and down as thoroughly as I had. My son Jack came home from soccer practice, we sat down for dinner, and I told him how Greg would have two boys now, just like us.

While I was washing the dishes, the phone rang. "Kurt, I've got a little situation here," Greg said. I had noticed over the years that he occasionally tried to appropriate doctorspeak when we'd had a few drinks in us. One day he told me that he wished he'd gone to med school, but now, at forty, all he could do was relish my stories. I chuckled for a second at his word choice because "situation" is the euphemism we doctors use to describe a complicated scenario.

Both boys had had near-perfect Apgar scores, and Lukas, the older twin, had breastfed a couple times. But Ezekiel was proving a harder case. He dozed and lolled all day long. Then an hour earlier, when Greg had picked him up and tried to burp him, he had thrown up all over Greg's shoulder. As Greg looked down at the mess, he saw that the vomit was green. It didn't feel right to him, and he'd raced out of the room to the nurse's stand with the green vomit dripping down his shirt to dial me.

Greg told me the nurse had rushed the baby to the hospital's NICU. We kept in touch by text, and within half an hour Greg told me that green fluid was being drained from Ezekiel through a nasogastric tube. Thirty minutes later, as he sat looking at Ezekiel's heart monitor, Greg saw his other son, Lukas, being wheeled into the NICU. Lukas's glucose level had been running in the low range of normal all day, and suddenly it had plummeted.

Greg texted me that both boys' vital signs and temperatures were normal, and the neonatal nurse practitioner on duty that evening had tried to calm him. Suddenly, Greg said, Ezekiel passed gas so loudly that for a moment he assumed the culprit was the nurse standing beside him. The nurse checked the boy's diaper. He had pooped for the first time. Everyone applauded and reassured Greg that Ezekiel's intestines were surely now working well and they just had to suction the bile that had backed up over the course of the day. They did an X-ray, which showed big air bubbles in Ezekiel's stomach, and the nurse practitioner reassured him that the suction would clear these out, too.

I related all this to Alison, who already knew from overhearing the conversation what must be done. An intestinal blockage could lead to perforation or the necrosis of Ezekiel's intestine. The only sure way to determine if there was such a blockage was to do a contrast study, and it should not wait until nine the next morning—when Greg had been told that the hospital's radiology team would be available. Waiting could mean compromising his intestine or possibly even death.

I called Greg immediately. "You can't wait until morning," I said. "I am going to be very frank with you: the delay could cause bigger problems. I'll arrange for emergency transport." I didn't know if his insurance would cover the ambulance ride, and I didn't tell him what a delay in diagnosing a blockage could mean. We would deal with the details later.

At two a.m., an ambulance carrying Ezekiel arrived at Children's National. The radiology imaging team whisked him away, and a NICU nurse walked Greg to what would become his sons' NICU room for the next seven weeks.

Dr. Tony Sandler was on call that night, and he walked into the room thirty minutes later and broke the news to Greg: the contrast study had showed a blockage and surgery was urgent. Greg signed the papers and watched Dr. Sandler dash off toward the operating rooms. I went to the OR to watch the procedure. To this day I still can't get enough of surgery, and I am always looking for an excuse to pop in.

Twenty minutes later, Dr. Mikael Petrosyan, a surgical fellow at the time, looked in and saw a dazed father staring into space. He asked a nurse for the details of the case.

When he entered the room, Greg assumed the worst and looked up in defeat. "Look," Dr. Petrosyan told him, seeking to console him, "this is what we do. This is what we do." Then he turned around and left.

Greg told me later that Dr. Petroysan's declaration—five words from a total stranger—did for him what a great coach's halftime speech does for a struggling team: *This is what we do*. It was so simple and matter-of-fact. He kept repeating it to himself, and it gave him the confidence to believe that things might be all right.

And in the end it was. Ezekiel's bowel was twisted and blocked, but it had not yet died for lack of blood flow. He responded well to the untwisting of his bowel, and at last blood flow to the intestine could commence. Dr. Sandler then configured the intestine so as to make sure the malrotation would not happen again.

As I watched, I couldn't help but marvel at the long arc of pediatric health issues. Only ten years earlier, Alison had rushed me to Georgetown University Hospital with a bowel obstruction. I ended up having surgery, and the general surgeon (my close friend Dr. Steve Evans, whom I had met while in training up in Boston) actually called in a pediatric surgeon from Children's National, Dr. Phil Guzzetta, to offer his perspective on this distinctly pediatric condition. It turned out I had been carrying a pediatric abnormality like Ezekiel's around inside me for fifty-four years.

The circumstances of Ezekiel's care are repeated hundreds of times a month in the United States. Newborns with complications can lose critical hours getting their conditions diagnosed or treated at a lower-level NICU. The knowledge that a sophisticated contrast study, and not merely an X-ray, is needed to determine a blockage is pretty basic at a children's hospital. But lower-level NICUs at nonspecialized hospitals, even established ones, don't perform the same volume of pediatric cases and don't tend to get the hard ones referred to them, so they don't develop the same sixth sense for conditions and procedures.

Those three aspects—around-the-clock access to specialists, and the greater volume and complexity of the cases they see—fundamentally distinguish NICUs at pediatric hospitals from most others. What upsets me is how few people know this. The general population—including thoughtful and cautious people like Greg and Alicia—assumes that high-level care is available around the clock at well-respected delivery centers with NICUs. But that is far from the case. Only Level IV NICUs may have around-the-clock access to pediatric specialists. In fact, a new rating system for hospitals is being developed based on their resources for neonatal surgical care. Championed by the American College of Surgeons, the new rating system highlights the importance of the immediate link between a NICU and a well-staffed pediatric hospital with surgical and anesthesia capability. This new rating system should enable parents like Greg and Alicia to know what a hospital NICU's capabilities are in the event of a severe crisis.

According to the March of Dimes, the number of preterm births as a percentage of all births has declined from 12.3 percent in 2003 to 11.4 percent in 2013. But that still means close to half a million babies are born in the United States each year with NICU-worthy complications. Approximately 3 percent of babies are born into extreme prematurity. People are starting families later in life, and reproductive technologies are making once-challenging pregnancies possible, but these pregnancies can be complicated or precarious. Beyond that, built into fetal life are complex biological processes that will inevitably result in a certain number of difficult cases. The logical deduction is that a state-of-the-art NICU staffed with experienced professionals is critical. We had that at Children's National.

But what we didn't have in place was a system to enable us to collaborate seamlessly with hospitals and birthing centers across the region, to eliminate the confusion Greg and Alicia faced. Together with our chief medical officer, Dr. David Wessel, I recruited one of the nation's leaders in neonatal network development, Dr. Robin Steinhorn. Like many of her peers, Dr. Steinhorn had found her calling in medical school. Just as med students who are drawn to pediatrics self-select, neonatologists often experience a triggering event. Babies inspire them with an intensity that is a cut above the norm. Dr. Steinhorn joined us in October 2015 and set out to help us build our hospital into the go-to center for NICUs and delivery rooms across the region.

"I am a lung specialist within the field of neonatology," Dr. Steinhorn told me as we walked through her hushed NICU one recent morning before dawn. "I focus on how the blood vessels work in the lungs. Yesterday we admitted a tiny baby born at another hospital who had been there for many weeks. She was doing okay, but her progress was static—she wasn't gaining sufficient weight to be discharged. So the NICU where she was contacted us, and we arranged transport. After half a day of observation and study of her records, we determined that she was masking, through her sheer strength and fight, very severe pulmonary hypertension."

In a perfect world, we would have caught this a lot earlier and jump-started the baby's development much sooner. NICUs at children's hospitals don't necessarily employ better neonatologists; they just see more problems and see them more often. Be it cardiologists monitoring newborn babies' hearts, otolaryngologists working on hearing issues, or behavioral therapists, specialty centers across the country have the pediatric infrastructure in place to track and treat a newborn with problems until all the medical issues are fully conquered. This can take months or years, but having those relationships in place from the get-go is essential.

Dr. Steinhorn and her peers in the region are working to improve coordination and communication among hospitals to bring access to high-level care to all babies, not just those whose parents are savvy enough or lucky enough to end up at a NICU at a specialized center. Telemedicine is a big part of it, and Dr. Steinhorn is working with several hospitals to get images and test results transferred to experts at our NICU in real time, so that doctors can discuss their findings and support babies even without relocating them.

"There is a resolve at neonatology specialty centers nationwide to reach out to communities and really bring our expertise to them," Robin told me when we discussed her vision for getting more babies the specialized care they need. "As a nation, we underfund neonatology. If a mother delivers at a hospital with a lower-level NICU, she should have immediate and seamless access to our level of care. We serve as that final stop on the continuum. There is no problem that is too difficult for us to take on and to improve. Confusing cases should be brought to us instantly using digital technology, so that we can examine X-rays in partnership with neonatologists at regional hospitals and consult with them."

Dr. Steinhorn's vision of a nervous system of NICUs with hubs and satellites working together in this way would have spared Greg and Alicia their tough night and given Ezekiel a chance to go home much sooner. If this vision materializes, future parents will never have to go through what they experienced. Babies will be born at a hospital that is part of a cohesive neonatal network, eliminating the gaps through which thousands fall each year. One obstacle is that NICUs are strong profit centers for most hospitals that have them, so the current system of hospital reimbursements works against this collaborative model.

Despite this challenge, our current efforts focus on making it easy for other institutions to collaborate with us. Dr. Steinhorn and her team have been working with local and regional hospitals to rotate our neonatologists into their NICUs and to regularly visit other NICUs in the area for conferences and collaborative sessions. The resulting camaraderie and shared commitment help to mitigate some of the conflicts surrounding transfers. A difficult case can be identified and sent to us quickly, before a crisis occurs. Or our doctors can be consulted and the infant can stay put. Because we invest in a top-notch transport system that is ready to go 24/7 on a few minutes' notice, we are confident about the transition.

Recently I was taking one of our donors for a tour of the hospital. We were walking through the NICU when she tugged on my arm and pulled me over to watch as a nurse practitioner threaded a catheter through a baby's tiny vein toward the heart to administer specialized intravenous nutrition. I knew this nurse practitioner was the go-to for tricky intravenous access. I told my guest that even within our NICU, there were unique talents for certain difficult tasks. I walked her through our vision of a network of NICUs with a hub, telemedicine, and regional collaboration.

She shook her head and marveled, then grew visibly concerned. "I'm about to become a grandmother for the first time, Kurt," she said. "And I don't think my daughter has any idea about any of this. I'm going to call her tonight."

I laughed, thinking to myself, *I haven't become so much a CEO as preacher, dedicated to educating parents about the value of pediatric specialization.* And sometimes I was just the guy who picked up the phone, as I did for Greg. Ezekiel was lucky, but no parent or child should have to depend on a stroke of luck to get the sort of neonatal care that can make all the difference.

CHAPTER 24:
Brains

If your child is one of the 25.5 million kids in the United States who will make a visit to the emergency room this year, he or she is likely to leave with more than a physical scar. I sure did. I was seven years old, standing with my five-year-old brother on a sand pile on a construction site. We were playing King of the Hill, and somehow I tripped and fell face-first into the scattered cinder blocks below. I tried to break my fall, but I gashed my right hand on a cinder block. I felt the blood before I felt the pain. When I looked up at my hand, I saw blood shooting everywhere.

My brother had learned the word *emergency* from some television show. He looked at all the blood and shouted, "Emergency! Emergency!"

I got up and ran down the street toward our home, my brother trailing a few feet behind and calling out to the neighborhood, "Emergency! Emergency!"

I can recall few specifics of my treatment in the ER, and I don't remember getting stitched up. But a general sense of discomfort and fear has stuck with me, and I do vividly recall the sights and sounds of that foreign place. Yellow curtains separated the beds, and adults groaned as they were pushed past on gurneys. These memories, more sensory than incidental, show how powerful and enduring a child's experience of the ER can be.

Years later I was fortunate to train under Dr. Marty Eichelberger, the Brazilian-born trauma specialist I wrote about in Chapter 14. He and Dr. Joseph Wright were leading a nationwide revolution in pediatric emergency care, developing protocols and minimum hospital standards for child-specific equipment. I learned from them the value of differentiating emergency care for kids, and that treatment at a children's hospital offers several distinct advantages. Pediatric doctors and nurses pay more careful attention to how a child's size and weight will dictate the size of their breathing tube or a dosage of anesthesia or painkiller. Beyond that, children's hospitals foster an atmosphere that aims to calm kids' nerves. We didn't think a lot about child psychology when I first started in medicine, but we now understand that severe stress can seriously impede healing.

When I became CEO, I suspected I shouldn't touch a department that was treating more than three hundred children per day and functioning so well. But it bugged me how little people realized what we were up to. When their kid broke an arm or twisted an ankle playing soccer, most parents rushed them to the *closest* ER. How could we get the word out that the best long-term outcome depended on getting not to the *closest* ER but to the most *child-focused* one? Years of experience on the messy front lines of emergency care had taught me that a child treated at a pediatric emergency room, seen and cared for by pediatric doctors and nurses, has a much higher likelihood of long-term health and welfare.

I started to think that my most important job might be not to improve what we were doing so much as to educate parents. I gave speeches at schools and talked to whoever would listen at dinner parties. On radio interviews and even at the gym, at playgrounds and at my own kids' sports events, I urged parents to come up with an emergency plan and to find the nearest pediatric ER. My buzz phrase became "brains and bones." Children's hospitals understand and treat concussions and fractures with such a keen understanding of children's unique biology and psychology that the long-term result is generally far superior.

Until my sons and their friends began playing competitive sports in high school, I didn't fully realize how common concussions are now among kids—and how important it is to treat them properly. One Friday night not too long ago, I sat in the stands with my son Jack and my best friends, Ted and Francesca, watching their son Kyle quarterback his high school football team on a long touchdown drive. My friends were proud of their son for rising to the starter's job, though Francesca had expressed concern to me about the violent nature of the sport. I told her the risks were real, but on this day I couldn't help but get into the swing of things, and I cheered as Kyle sprinted for a touchdown.

"I never thought I'd say this," Francesca half whispered to me, "but I can finally see how complex football is. I thought it was just a bunch of boys running into each other. But I'm proud of how intelligently he seems to be running his team."

I shared her pride and was enjoying the spirit of the game until halfway through the second quarter, when Kyle started acting oddly on the field. He walked clumsily and struggled to grasp the play signals his coach was relaying from the sideline. At one point, he forgot to join the huddle to share the game plan with his team for the next play. And yet he kept completing pass after pass, orchestrating a march down the field that would tie the game in the fourth quarter. His behavior suggested that he had suffered a concussion, but I had been watching closely and had not seen him take a hit. Even when the brain is injured, it can still function, and Kyle's football skills and instincts had become almost second nature.

He deceived even me, and I should have known better than to fall for it, for a concussed brain is particularly vulnerable to further injury given its weakened condition.

His mother fidgeted beside me. Finally she grabbed my arm and squeezed it tightly. "Kurt, you have to go down there—something is really wrong with him!" she said loudly. "Something is really wrong!"

Ted looked at me, and we both raced down the stands. The fans erupted just as we reached the team— Kyle had thrown a touchdown pass. We met him on the sideline, where his teammates were patting him on the shoulder, but then he sat down on a bench looking into space. As we squatted in front of him, I was certain he had suffered a concussion.

"What's the score?" he kept asking. An ambulance was parked at the other end of the field, the EMT leaning against it. I motioned for him to bring the ambulance over. Kyle was disoriented and could not remember the important events of the game. This kind of confusion is one of the red flags that indicates the need for emergency care. While not all kids have to be transported to the emergency department after a concussion, when they exhibit disorientation, it's better to get them to the hospital.

"How's he look?" an assistant coach asked, as Kyle's father and I tried to assess his condition. "Our defense is going to hold. We've got to get him back on the field to win this thing!"

I wanted to turn around and slug the guy.

As the EMT prepared Kyle for the ride on the stretcher, I asked him where his protocol required him to transport the young man.

"The nearest hospital," he said.

That wasn't the answer I wanted. "Let's drive him down to Children's ourselves," I said to Ted, who nodded firmly and rushed off to get his van. I rode in the back with Kyle, while Ted and Francesca sat up front.

I called ahead to Dr. Gerry Gioia, our concussion specialist, who was on call most Friday nights during football season. Dr. Gioia put Kyle through a detailed neuropsychological exam, assessing his cognitive functioning (attention, memory) and balance, and the ER doctor gave him a standard physical exam (vision, motor strength, reflexes) to identify subtle motor weakness. There were multiple signs that Kyle's brain functioning was critically impaired—poor memory, slowed speech, and an array of postconcussion symptoms including a headache, fatigue, sensitivity to light, poor balance, and difficulty concentrating.

It took Dr. Gioia and his team three weeks to help Kyle to fully heal.

They put a rehabilitation plan in place specifically designed for an active teenager. They instructed him to shut down all physical and cognitive activities and ordered bed rest for almost a week. After that first week, they gradually reintroduced schoolwork, followed by a little social activity (friends), and after two weeks, physical activity. Dr. Gioia outlined a school support plan for his parents and teachers and coached his parents through its implementation. A well-calibrated and individualized rehabilitation plan is fundamental to long-term recovery from a concussion. It is astonishing how often this is simply not understood.

Had Kyle gone back into the game, as scores of adolescents do every week under similar circumstances, he would have risked a second concussion—a potentially lethal event. Had he not been administered such a thorough and lengthy recovery regimen with its careful reintegration into daily teenage life, his brain would not have healed as well, and he might have suffered long-term consequences. The problems sometimes crop up decades later, long after any record remains of the original accident.

As a pediatric neuropsychologist, Dr. Gioia spearheaded a new treatment algorithm for childhood concussions, emphasizing the brain's developmental stages. He is quick to point out the many differences between a six- and a fourteen-year-old brain. As a result of his research, medical providers around the country have a new set of tools to test children's brain functioning after a concussion and new protocols to treat an array of injuries. Familiarity with children's brains is as fundamental to the treatment plan for adolescent athletes like Kyle as for wobbly young ice skaters who take a hard fall.

No tissue is torn in a concussion, but as the brain sloshes around in its surrounding fluid, chemicals are fired off at abnormal rates. The cells (axons) that connect regions of the brain through electrical currents are stretched, rendering the network dysfunctional for a period of time. The brain's energy is significantly depleted as well. Neuroscientists sometimes speak of concussion as a software injury. With more severe brain injuries, you can see actual tissue damage on CT and MRI scans. Concussions distort the brain's neurochemical "software" more than its structural "hardware," but a prolongation of this condition can result in long-term damage to both.

The abnormal electrical and chemical activity triggered by a concussion results in a host of symptoms. Some are physical (headaches, difficulty focusing, dizziness, and balance issues), some cognitive (trouble concentrating and remembering things), and some emotional (irritability, excessive response to stress, and sleep problems). Fortunately, the brain has a natural ability to repair itself over time. But you need to know what to do to make it possible. The first step is to appreciate that many childhood concussions are never diagnosed or treated. The second is to recognize that treatment is necessary and will take time. The brain needs to rest so that it can heal. This means that it must have less stimulus—no phones and social media, less social interaction, fewer demands. If you want your child to heal, you have to speak to their teachers and explain the need for time out. Then you need to carefully and slowly resume as much normal daily activity as the child can tolerate.

While the principles of pediatric concussion treatment are consistent, the plan differs significantly for the six-year-old, the twelve-year-old, and the sixteen-year-old, as we must take the developmental differences in these different brains into account. To illustrate the importance of a precise, developmentally based approach to treating children with brain trauma, Dr. Gioia told me about James, a six-year-old boy he'd recently treated. James fell down the stairs at home and suffered a series of sharp blows to the head. His parents took him to a general emergency department, and after an interminable wait, he was seen and sent home with vague instructions to take it easy over the next few days. When his headaches continued over the course of several weeks and his behavior became erratic, his parents took him to an outpatient clinic. Neither place seriously factored into its diagnosis or treatment the fact that he was six years old. No one sat down with his parents to establish a clear plan for him to rest, recover, and slowly return to normal activity on a step-by-step basis.

"You have to focus on the age of the child and on the family as a unit," Dr. Gioia told me, "so you really have in some ways two patients."

Pediatric specialists have a clear understanding of how a concussion affects a child's developing cognitive, social, and emotional functioning. There are two main differences in how concussions are treated in the developing brain. First, if an image (CT scan or MRI) is necessary to rule out bleeding, intracranial pressure, swelling, or other structural changes, the physician must be trained to recognize different developmental benchmarks. A four-year-old brain looks nothing like a forty-four-year-old brain. Pediatric practitioners know how to handle distressed kids and reduce the anxiety around the use of a CT scanner or an MRI machine. (Experience working with kids is critical to setting them at ease.) Second, the manifestations of a concussion in a child or adolescent can look different, and children will describe their symptoms differently. Most young kids do not understand how to explain dizziness or fogginess or even a headache, let alone concentration problems or irritability—all common symptoms. The pediatric provider knows to modify his or her language and understands what is normal and abnormal as the measures change over time.

"Certain aspects of behavioral and emotional control are affected when a child's brain is injured," Dr. Gioia explained to me. "Pediatric specialists have a sliding scale of development ingrained in our heads that adult specialists just don't have."

A six-year-old is not all that much in control to begin with, but when James went home from the emergency department, he played too hard too soon. This premature return to his normal, kinetic way of life intensified his symptoms. He cried much more and grew enraged at the smallest provocation. No one had counseled his parents on how to pace his resumed play. His mother then swung in the opposite direction and became overprotective, but that too can have adverse consequences. Failure to calibrate James's recovery had triggered additional brain trauma, and he ended up needing physical therapy and psychological treatment to fully heal.

The brain injury spectrum in kids is wide and quirky. Dr. Gioia and his staff aggressively engage parents as co-caregivers and see it as their responsibility to educate them about their child's distinct recovery needs. They calibrate reentry into the school day, not just into sports activities. Caregivers and doctors who have not been trained in this developmental approach usually focus primarily on a return to the playing field, but a careful calibration of the school day is even more fundamental. The rigors and multiple sensory and emotional demands of thinking and interacting in a classroom can harm the wounded brain.

If I were king for a day, every city in the United States would have a pediatric ER with the tools to address children's unique biological, neurological, and psychological needs. But getting this message out in my own community, and even among my friends, is challenge enough.

CHAPTER 25:
Bones

When my son Jack was about ten years old, all he wanted to do was play soccer. He played after school and all day on weekends and would have kept at it all night if we'd let him. He was a very active boy, so like many parents, we encouraged him to play a lot of soccer to run out his energy. Soccer has become the best friend of parents nationwide. It keeps a lot of boys and girls out of trouble in the United States and around the world.

But one day Jack complained about knee pain. Over the course of several weeks, the problem became more pronounced, until one Saturday he had to come out of a game because the pain was so intense. After the game, he could barely walk to the car with me. I took him straight to the Children's National ER. The pediatric orthopedic surgeon on call that day, Dr. John Lovejoy, didn't think there was anything structurally wrong with Jack's knee and found no swelling. Yet I could tell from his expression that something concerned him.

"But?" I asked, after a pause.

"I think we'd better take a closer look at things," he said. "We're seeing more and more growth plate issues in kids your age, Jack. Do you know what that means?"

Jack shook his head, and Dr. Lovejoy went on to explain how growth plates work. An injury to the growth plate, he said, can distort how a bone grows and complicate the functioning of a joint. Any damage to the plates needs to be addressed as part of the healing process. He recommended an MRI of Jack's knees. I thought this might be overkill but didn't want to contradict him.

An MRI is an unpleasant experience under any circumstances, and even adults have a hard time being confined in such a tight and cold space for so long. At most pediatric hospitals, the child's psychology drives the experience. A Child Life specialist talked to Jack and kept him engaged and calm during the hour-long procedure. As a result, he didn't require sedation. Our MRI room had been painted to look like an underwater submarine, so he was distracted by the sea creatures floating around him and was actually excited to get inside the submarine. The warmth and calmness of the room made the technology feel less intimidating, even to me. I could tell Jack was at ease, despite the shock of discovering that he might have a more serious problem than we'd imagined.

The MRI showed that Jack had inflammation around his growth plates. Only a well-practiced pediatric radiologist and pediatric orthopedist together would have spotted it—inflammation is hard to detect on an MRI. Luckily, there was no sign of permanent damage or what we call necrosis—tissue death. Dr. Lovejoy told us that the plates would recover with good rest, physical therapy, and a more limited play schedule. The normal prescription—ice, Advil, and a few days off—could have resulted in permanent damage once Jack resumed playing soccer. The findings on the MRI were very subtle, and having a pediatric specialist interpret them made all the difference to Jack's long-term athletic career and his ability to walk pain free.

The father in me feels the urge to give my "brains and bones" speech every chance I get. Parents sometimes call to tell me that they need to see a pediatric orthopedic surgeon because their child's initial visit to a general emergency department resulted in fracture care that did not account for growth plates, leading to complications and the need for more surgery.

Children's broken arms and ankles, femurs and tibias are best treated by a pediatric orthopedic surgeon, who will focus on getting the plates back in line so that growth can proceed once the bone has healed without long-term consequences. So much of a child's medical life plays out in pediatric emergency care. Innovative treatment can remedy a child's emergency in such a way that, as fifty- and sixty-year-olds, they will have grateful rather than traumatic memories—and fewer secondary effects from their childhood injury.

Ironically, a visit to a children's ER often results in less treatment as the better strategy. Dr. Stephen Teach, a long-standing emergency doctor at our hospital, points to a recent case where doing less yielded better results for the child than the more aggressive course of action proposed by the community ER center the boy had originally visited.

A five-year-old boy had a low-grade fever, a growing rash, and one Saturday morning was suddenly refusing to walk. His parents had watched his progress with concern and debated what to do. By the time he stopped walking, they were in a low-grade panic and brought him to the emergency room of a community hospital some fifty miles from downtown D.C. The ER doctors examined the boy and found that his hands, feet, and ankles were swollen. The rash, which was concentrated on his legs and buttocks, did not blanch when it was pressed. Several doctors conferred and agreed that that suggested vasculitis. When accompanied by a fever, it seemed to indicate a severe blood infection. If this was the case, the risks included loss of fingers, toes, limbs, and even death.

They took the child to their resuscitation room, administered oxygen, and hooked him up to an IV to dose him with fluids and antibiotics. They began an intravenous medication to support his blood pressure, although the blood pressure, perfusion (blood flow), and mental status were normal. The doctor in charge then called the emergency department at Children's National to request emergency transport by helicopter.

One hour later Dr. Teach was in the ER, where he could hear the helicopter approaching the helipad atop our building. Dr. Teach had spoken several times with the referring physicians and was ready to pounce. When the transport team whisked the boy in, he and his colleagues ran through the checklist of symptoms they had been discussing.

Then they began to study the rash. An emergency nurse said she had seen similar characteristics on a young girl a week earlier. It was indeed red and nonblanching, but the team recognized it as Henoch-Schönlein purpura, an uncommon and relatively benign form of vasculitis. The child was disconnected from the oxygen and intravenous lines and discharged an hour later with pain medication and told to follow up with his primary care provider the following day.

Less is more—sometimes in a big way. Every procedure involves risks, and a doctor's job is to weigh them. Is it wiser to be safe in case of an outside possibility, or to watch and monitor and spare a child unnecessary intervention? The training and experience of pediatric professionals often leads to better outcomes precisely because of what they elect not to do. At nonpediatric centers, overtreatment can sometimes do as much damage as mistreatment.

In a perfect world, I wouldn't have to be a preacher, and the data would speak for themselves. Fifteen percent of all emergency departments reported critical pediatric equipment as missing; 69 percent of the EDs nationwide see an average of less than 14 pediatric patients per day; and 85 percent of all EDs are configured as general EDs with no separation of children. ERs at children's centers treat hundreds of kids a day. The numbers speak for themselves. And there is a deeper medical logic, too. Pediatric emergency specialists who are familiar and comfortable with treating children order fewer unnecessary CT scans for head injury, fewer unnecessary blood tests for asthma, and fewer unnecessary antibiotics for viral infections. Unnecessary diagnostic tests and therapies pose a risk both to individual patients and to the community at large. (The overprescription of antibiotics has fostered the development of antibiotic-resistant strains of bacteria.) They also represent a waste of medical resources and unnecessary health care costs.

At Children's National, we have been actively working to decrease the rates of chest X-rays for asthma and diagnostic testing for low-risk patients. We reduced CT scans for head injury by 40 percent by supporting clinical decisions with careful examination of patients' electronic health records. We are working with other children's hospitals in an effort to make similar reductions at their emergency departments. Collaborating with ERs at Ann and Robert H. Lurie Children's Hospital of Chicago, Children's Hospital Colorado, Cincinnati Children's Hospital Medical Center, and the Children's Hospital of Philadelphia, we have created a registry of all emergency department visits for the last three years. Together we provide report cards to more than three hundred physicians each month, drawn from patient feedback on pain management and the duration of ER visits. This national web is growing more seamless and fruitful every year. The new frontier of pediatric medicine is a place of medical innovation, but it also involves a growing level of cooperation and data analysis nationally.

In the meantime, I advise parents to ask their pediatricians to pose two key questions to their ERs of choice as they formulate their pediatric emergency plan: How many children do you treat in your ER every year? Do you have pediatric ER specialists staffing the ER department? Parents should also determine the accessibility (in terms of both location and insurance) of the closest child-specialized emergency center. You will want to know the answers to these questions before the next emergency occurs.

CHAPTER 26:

The Science of Pain

I always suspected that Dr. Randolph's favorite patient was Lonnie, a round-faced boy from Baltimore with a faulty lymphatic system, a side effect of which was chronic swelling in his leg, pelvis, and abdomen. The underlying cause of the disease was incurable, and the fluid buildup and backlog made Lonnie's body a magnet for infection. We had to operate on him regularly to excise these infections and cysts because antibiotics alone could not eliminate them entirely. Dr. Randolph became, in some sense, Lonnie's personal antibiotic. He must have cut into Lonnie more than thirty times. He was Lonnie's palliative care doctor, too, as not even the strongest painkillers could give Lonnie total relief from his pain. Only his scalpel could.

Thanks to his lion's heart and his empowering family, Lonnie plodded on. I assisted Dr. Randolph on yet another excision and wondered, *How much of this can he take? How many times can he bear coming in here and being cut into?*

In his teenage years, Lonnie gained fame among the doctors and nurses. We tend to remember patients based on their sense of humor and urge to banter with us despite the circumstances. Like Casey (whom we met in Chapter 17), Lonnie brought a precocious charisma to his conversations with adults. Perhaps unsurprisingly, his chats with Dr. Randolph centered on sports. Lonnie loved baseball. He and Dr. Randolph would tease each other about their respective favorite teams, the Atlanta Braves and the Baltimore Orioles. Lonnie usually got the upper hand, because he was so knowledgeable about the players and the team's statistics.

Dr. Randolph maintained an uncanny optimism in front of patients and colleagues alike. Rarely did I glimpse despair or heartbreak. But one Saturday afternoon when I was on call, I peered through a crack in his office door and spotted him at his desk. The surgery offices were eerily quiet on weekends, and I was surprised to see the light on. Dr. Randolph was a renowned letter writer, and he would spend hours spinning handwritten notes to parents and patients. I craved to know what made him tick, and I sensed he had not heard me, so I tiptoed closer to study what he was like when no one was watching.

As I zeroed in on him, I grew concerned. He looked despondent, even grim. I had rarely seen his face not radiating joy or optimism. He also had great posture, but now he sat slumped on his chair, rubbing his eyes with the palms of his hands.

My voyeurism embarrassed me, so I coughed to signal my presence and pushed his door open. "You look like you had a rough night of drinking," I wisecracked, knowing full well that he was a devoted teetotaler who believed that even one drink could undermine his performance as a surgeon.

"Lonnie's back," he said. This must have been the umpteenth time Lonnie, now in his early twenties, had come in for surgery. "I just don't know what kind of life this young man has to look forward to. He can't even play sports anymore. I don't know if I can keep faking this happy face with him and his family. We are hitting the end of the road."

Dr. Randolph's candor and emotion stunned me. I said something to console him, then looked at the floor, wondering what he would decide to do.

The next day, as we examined Lonnie together, Dr. Randolph was all sun and optimism again. He told Lonnie we would fix him up and get him moving in the right direction. But as we walked out of the room, his face abruptly gave in again; sadness filled his eyes, and the bravado evaporated. That day I realized that part of our job as pediatric specialists was to fake it.

And faking it was the part of the job I hated most.

When I was interviewing to be CEO of the hospital that Dr. Randolph had helped build, I thought back to Lonnie and to Victoria, and I decided I would do everything in my power to ensure we never saw another Lonnie or Victoria again. Joe Robert and I regularly asked ourselves and our team members the same questions: How can we systematically reduce pain in children—or even eliminate it? How much more progress could children make if pain were not a factor? How can we reduce the use of opioid-based painkillers and make the war against childhood pain one of our core missions?

A main objective of the Sheikh Zayed Institute was to find a way to measure pain in children. We could take a patient's pulse or blood pressure and measure their blood cell types and counts. We could administer varying doses of medication perfectly calibrated to a child's body weight. But we still had to rely on the antiquated pain scoring system—happy faces and sad faces—to gauge what they were feeling. It was woefully inadequate because it was purely subjective and could not be compared across patients. And when it came to babies and nonverbal or autistic children, it had almost no value. Research was showing that babies and infants experience pain differently, suggesting that the typical therapies might not be effective.

Sometimes I felt embarrassed having to ask a child which face fit her level of discomfort. With all these amazing things, all this incredible technology around us, the best we could do was hold up a chart with smiley faces on it to understand how a child felt. A more precise and scientific way of measuring pain would lead to new treatments, we reasoned, and that was another significant objective. Understanding pain types and levels precisely would be the first step toward establishing a new approach to pediatric pain management, which would in turn open a frontier for new treatments across a range of conditions, as pain—not biology—so often limited our options.

Dr. Julie Finkel, an anesthesiologist at Children's National who was also doing pain research at the National Institutes of Health (NIH) up the road in Bethesda, became our solution. Dr. Finkel's professional dream was to measure pain accurately and to use this knowledge to determine whether a certain treatment or intervention was effective. If you couldn't measure pain, she reasoned, you couldn't truly address it.

Dr. Finkel was making great progress in her lab, and we wanted to make her work a central part of the Sheikh Zayed Institute. The institute's mantra was "to make surgery more precise, less invasive, and pain free," and I felt the time had come to focus on that last, most difficult piece. We decided to form what we called the Pain Center within the institute and to empower Dr. Finkel and her colleagues to try to solve the riddle of pain.

Dr. Zena Quezado, Dr. Finkel's research partner at the NIH, was the chief of anesthesia there and a pediatric anesthesiologist to boot. She had been the regular anesthesiologist for Joe Robert's neurosurgeon at the NIH, which I took as a good omen. Together Dr. Finkel and Dr. Quezado brought their research enterprise from the NIH to our hospital and began innovative studies to measure pain using patients' own nervous system and its response to different stimuli.

A couple of years after they joined us, Dr. Finkel invited me to come see the technology she and her team had developed. I was used to getting calls from our researchers with their latest discoveries, and while I appreciated their innate enthusiasm for science, I was often underwhelmed: the results didn't always pan out with actual patients in clinical trials.

Dr. Finkel's breakthrough was to use the pupil's response to assess the presence and intensity of pain. Walking up the stairs to her laboratory, I remembered how I had been taught back in medical school to examine the eye's pupillary response to assess the responsiveness of the nervous system and the brain, and even the patient's level of consciousness. It was a routine part of any neurologic exam—shining a light into each eye to gauge the size of the pupil and determine how quickly it constricted. An uneven response, or a pupil that was larger than the other, or dilation of both, meant something serious was going on. Every doctor knew this, but I couldn't see how it had anything to do with pain. I had performed the exam myself thousands of times on children—was it possible I had been missing something so essential?

Entering the lab, I could feel Dr. Finkel's excitement. As soon as she saw me, she grabbed her smartphone. I wasn't quite sure what she was doing, but then she showed me the small attachment, a camera that had been adapted to measure the pupil. I began to get a sense of where this was going. She described how the pupil was responsive to different types of pain stimuli and said that its dilation could be measured and quantified. Her lab had demonstrated a direct correlation between the degree of pain and the extent of dilation. She had found a way to measure pain and—indirectly—the ability of medications and therapies to alleviate it.

This is the Holy Grail of pediatric medicine! I thought to myself. *What wouldn't I give to put this smartphone in Joe Robert's hands?*

As Dr. Finkel went through a prototype examination, the simplicity of the device and its use for infants, children, and even adults became instantly clear. She showed me a video in which she delivered a stimulus with a tiny electrical output to a volunteer and measured with her camera what happened to his pupil. After watching a number of videotape demonstrations, I felt confident we were well on the way to finally being able to measure pain. This would unlock our ability to find new treatments and therapies designed for babies and children. We could finally throw that absurdly antiquated pain score chart out the window.

I sometimes feel my task as CEO is to create an environment in which research like this can happen and directly feed into clinical practice. Because of my pledge to Joe, but even more because I believe it can be truly transformative, I have made the growth of our Pain Center a priority. One of its first innovations, the use of gaming technology as therapy, is now an active tool in our war against pain. Developed in the bioengineering lab at the Sheikh Zayed Institute, gaming therapy uses video games to distract a child during therapy and then to expand the possibilities of therapy itself. If a child has nerve damage in her arm, for example, the pain team hooks her arm up to an electronic sleeve, and she plays a game similar to Angry Birds with that arm. The doctors monitor her movements on a computer, pushing her to expand her range of motion even while she loses herself in the game. Therapy becomes more effective even as it seemingly disappears.

Dr. Sean Alexander, one of several anesthesiologists who hang their scrubs at the Pain Center, has made gaming a central part of his work with recovering patients there. One of his most rewarding cases so far has been Rachel, a vivacious fourteen-year-old girl who broke a couple of bones in her left foot when she fell off a horse. She suffered damage to several ligaments in her foot and ankle area, and they were causing her pain even after the bones had healed. I visited her one day in the lab and watched as she played. I was struck by how she lost herself in the play. She reminded me of one of my sons playing a video game as she piloted a spaceship through the treacherous terrain of an unknown planet. I was witnessing not only the cutting edge of pediatric pain treatment but a realization of Joe Robert's vision of maintaining the integrity of childhood play inside the medical environment.

"Rachel developed what we call chronic regional pain syndrome," Dr. Alexander told me as we watched how rapt she was in her gaming therapy. "The orthopedic surgeons at her local hospital fixed her fracture, put her in a supportive cast, and sent her home. The real crisis started three months later. The pain returned and was beginning to affect her whole life. Over the next few months her sleep began to diminish and she began to have symptoms of depression. Rachel's pain began to take on a life of its own. Her pain syndrome was an example of how pain in one small spot can take over a child's life."

Dr. Alexander and other pain specialists instantly realized that the nerves in Rachel's foot and ankle had obviously been damaged, and because of chronic stimulation, an abnormal nerve-brain feedback loop had taken hold between her ankle and the pain centers of the brain. Her brain had become stuck in the pain rut that so many kids (and adults) slide into.

Rachel's pain was transforming her personality, something I saw in patients with alarming regularity. She missed school and was often irritable, and the smile her parents adored was flashing less frequently. She stayed in bed in the morning and refused to emerge. It got so bad that she would insist on wearing shorts on cold spring days. Putting on pants or jeans just hurt her too much, and she didn't dare touch her foot or ankle. The pain had reached its tentacles deep into her brain, and depression was taking hold.

Pain is not unlike muscle memory. Once a young person's body and mind learn to feel pain, it is difficult to break its patterns and rhythms. Those nerves learn certain pathways, and the feedback loop takes hold. Then the brain gets hardwired to experience pain because the nerves have learned a pattern of irritation.

Dr. Alexander and his team knew that only a multidimensional treatment program could undo these neurological habits. Sure, painkillers would be a part of the plan, but Rachel had been on painkillers for three months now. Not only were they contributing to her depression, but the pain was worsening because of the depression.

"We decided to double down on physical therapy and behavioral medicine and to add the gaming therapy to her plan," Dr. Alexander told me. "Gaming has been a very effective way of engaging her and getting her to do her PT with more dedication."

I watched as Rachel moved her foot and leg in a boot that controlled the spaceship's movements. She was steering with her legs, gasping and grunting at the close calls and daredevil moves she was making on screen. She was, without realizing it, reproducing the motion Dr. Alexander wanted her to relearn. This was no longer torture: Rachel was having fun and improving her condition at the same time. Dr. Alexander could adjust the game to incorporate different moves or angles and make movements more difficult without Rachel's realizing it.

The first month was touch and go, Rachel admitted. "At first I felt like they were tricking me, and I was stubborn," she told me. "I didn't want to give in and pretend I was cooperating with their trick."

She wanted to play, but she didn't want to play along. In the end, the lure of the gaming technology swayed her, and she slowly engaged with this new form of therapy. The Pain Center staff encouraged her mother, her father, and her two brothers to keep motivating her and to play along with her.

The second month provided Rachel and her family with a glimmer of hope. The physical therapist finally determined that she could break away from gaming and start doing real-life activities. At one PT session, she put on a pair of loose pants by herself. At another she slowly put on a sock. Both feats had been unimaginable until then.

With a little help, Rachel was regaining control of her brain—and her life. Pain had hijacked it, but now she was retraining it. This is the key point of gaming therapy: the brain can relearn what to feel and how to move without being shackled by pain. Halfway through her third month of therapy, Rachel's therapists heard the best news yet from her parents: her famous smile was slowly returning. Her body was loosening up, she was going out with friends once in a while, and she had started to tease her brothers back when they teased her.

"I don't think I would ever have regained this normal motion of my leg without gaming," Rachel told me. "My friends and I, people our age, this is what we do. Technology, the Internet, games. You're bringing our world to us here to help us recover."

The Pain Center is now adding more creative and innovative pain therapies like acupuncture, hypnosis, massage, and sleep therapy to the treatment plan for children. With cutting-edge treatments for pain, surgeons, cancer specialists, and physical therapists will be able to perform a broad range of interventions that will likely be more effective because they will involve less suffering.

Whenever I walk through the Pain Center and see Dr. Finkel's lab and the bioengineering research team working alongside Dr. Alexander and his colleagues, I think about the long-term view of the child that Dr. Randolph and Joe Robert were so passionate about. As more and more of my patients come back as adults for visits, they almost unanimously reflect more on the pain they experienced under our care than their interventions or even their brushes with death. Pain is what they most frequently ask us to address so that the kids of tomorrow won't have to endure the same suffering. Their requests, and the inspiration of patients like Lonnie and Victoria, are helping us turn a benefactor's vision of a pain-free future into a child's reality.

CHAPTER 27:

Peering into the Developing Brain

Toward the end of my surgical career, I met Shayna Kanfer in the most unusual of circumstances: she was inside her mother and was technically still a fetus. Shayna's mother had been referred to me by her obstetrician. Her baby had a large neck mass that was compressing her trachea and would prohibit her from breathing once the umbilical cord was cut. Even if, against all the odds, she made it to delivery, she would die soon afterward because her airway was blocked. We would have to operate before she was technically born to establish her breathing while she was still attached to her mother's umbilical cord.

The good news was that surgeons and obstetricians at the University of California at San Francisco (UCSF) had been using a new technique called the EXIT (ex utero intrapartum treatment) procedure. They had managed to keep a baby connected to the placenta during a C-section and partially deliver her to fix airway issues while she was still receiving oxygen from her mother through the umbilical cord.

I told the Kanfers that I would contact the UCSF doctors, and if I felt we could provide the resources and team to do the surgery, we would. Otherwise the family would have to relocate to San Francisco for the duration of the pregnancy.

One of the pleasures of pediatric medicine is the spirit of collegiality and collaboration that runs across children's hospitals. When I called the team in San Francisco to ask for insight and guidance, they gave it with enthusiasm. Based on their advice, we began putting together our own team, which would perform the EXIT procedure during a scheduled cesarean right around Christmas. The Kanfers understood the risks, and their confidence motivated us even more.

We built a playbook for the procedure and drilled as a team. We would perform a specialized C-section, making the uterine incision with a special type of stapler that cuts and staples at the same time. We would use special anesthesia and drugs to prevent uterine contractions, as they would otherwise disrupt umbilical circulation and cut off oxygen flow to the baby. We would monitor Shayna's progress closely while we delivered her partially from the womb to provide access to her mouth and airway. We would then perform a bronchoscopy and place an endotracheal tube while she was still connected to her mother's placenta.

We asked Shayna's mother to go on bed rest for several weeks: she was having intermittent contractions, and we wanted to make sure she didn't deliver prematurely. As Christmas approached, she was close to full term, and everybody canceled their vacation plans.

On the big day, the procedure got off to a good start. The obstetrical team did a beautiful job exposing the uterus and partially delivering the baby, and the cocktail of medications prevented premature contractions. We now had ten or fifteen minutes to place the endotracheal tube through Shayna's mouth. The tumor was so big, it distorted her face and neck, making the intubation difficult. We used the smallest available tube and corkscrewed it down past the tumor and into her lungs. When we were confident that it was in the right place and that oxygen would reach Shayna's lungs, we clamped the umbilical cord and cut it. The team delivered her the rest of the way, and the nurses and neonatologists took her to the NICU for the standard care.

Later that day I operated on Shayna again with a colleague, Dr. Lou Marmon, and we resected the cystic tumor from her neck. The size of the fluid-filled mass shocked me, but once we removed it, her face and neck slowly relaxed into a normal contour. Watching her distorted face recapture its newborn beauty was one of the most thrilling moments in my career.

This surgery taught me that the work of fetal specialists was directly linked to my own work as a surgeon. Their analysis and interventions were becoming as critical as NICU care. I came to see the period before and after birth as fluid and continuous in the life cycle, the fetus and the newborn meriting similar attention, care, and intervention.

In my own mental catalog, I rank Shayna's surgery as one of my most cutting-edge cases. But during and after the operation, we had been unable to assess the health of her brain. The technology didn't yet exist to measure fetal brain development. Shayna turned out great, but we had been lucky. My first fetal procedure left me fascinated with an organ we had neither focused on nor even touched. When the hospital decided to establish a new focus on brain health, this experience convinced me that we needed to go all the way back to the fetal brain. That was the real new frontier, back there in the womb.

Toward the end of my time as surgeon in chief, I inherited the case of a baby with a prenatal diagnosis that pointed to intestinal blockage. When the day came for the delivery, we addressed the obstruction but were surprised to discover a blockage of the esophagus that would require a second emergency procedure.

I will never forget the look in the parents' eyes when I rushed out to brief them prior to the second procedure.

"But what is the long-term impact?" the father asked as he struggled to process the news. "I mean, what typically have been the side effects for this sort of a case with regards to the brain?"

I was struck by his response. He was focused not on the immediate problems, as we were, but on the life this baby would grow into—and whether he might suffer from some form of mental impairment. It killed me that I could not look these parents in the eye and tell them that their son would be okay. I was confident the surgery itself would turn out well and had high hopes that so much anesthesia during the first hours of life would not damage the brain, but I couldn't provide them with absolute certainty.

That said, things were changing. Discoveries in other fields were producing stunning innovations that could well transform my own field. Genetics, immunotherapy, and fetal imaging all held the promise of reducing the future need for surgery.

A few years earlier, as surgeon in chief, I had participated in the hiring of Dr. Adre Du Plessis, a fetal neurologist. When we were trying to recruit him, he told us that over the next few decades we would be using advanced imaging to make prenatal diagnoses that would protect people from developing, later in life, diabetes, high blood pressure, and maybe even some cancers. When I became CEO, I learned that Dr. Du Plessis still did not have a centralized home for his team. His imaging group and specialists were dispersed around the hospital.

Dr. Du Plessis was half of a brilliant husband-and-wife team. His expertise as a clinical neuroscientist was complemented by the specialization of his wife, Dr. Catherine Limperopoulos, in advanced brain imaging. I felt that they deserved the best situation possible to undertake their mission to image the fetal brain and understand its precise functioning so that we could provide interventions and treatments just as we already could for fetal diaphragmatic hernias and heart murmurs. A young body needs every organ to function well for its owner to fully flourish, but the brain is the linchpin of all development. Brain stresses, including autism, genetic diseases, and more, had proven to be the least surmountable problem. Our new Fetal Medicine Institute would seek neurological treatments that could be applied during the fetal period, just as other children's hospitals, such as Cincinnati Children's Hospital, Children's Hospital of Philadelphia, and Texas Children's Hospital in Houston, were doing for other organs in the body.

We set about designing a space that addressed the needs of mothers, too. Our patients would be pregnant women, so everything from the examination rooms to the bathrooms had to be designed for their comfort and privacy. Because these were sensitive diagnoses with often heartbreaking prognoses, we wanted a place where our patients could take refuge and seek solace. We also wanted artwork for adults—not the kind that would stir up thoughts about babies.

Once the nine-month construction phase was finished, the fetal clinicians and researchers had a new home together. At the Fetal Medicine Institute, they began the urgent task of collecting and analyzing one of the world's largest databases of MRI images of normal fetal brains across the whole period of gestation. This database has allowed our center to detect the earliest deviations from the norm and to identify potential problems much earlier than we previously could. With her expert eye and cutting-edge imaging technology, Dr. Limperopoulos can spot the slightest departure from normal development in many regions of the brain. In her lab, every inch of space is devoted to technology—it looks like an air traffic control room, with dozens of screens and monitors. As I watched her work, I marveled at how different this is from what I was taught. I had seen ultrasound images of babies in utero and a few fetal MRIs, and radiologists had interpreted them for me, but it hadn't really hit me until now that you could scrutinize an individual organ like the brain, watch it develop almost in real time, and identify abnormalities long before the baby was born.

Dr. Limperopoulos pulled up an MRI scan for me that she had just done on a mother and her fetus. First she showed me the current image of the baby's brain at twenty-eight weeks; then she rolled a dial and tracked the brain's development backward, stopping at twenty weeks and then at fourteen to point out subtle blips. The brain was growing and enlarging, developing the folds and connections necessary for personality, speech, emotion, intelligence, and behavior right before my eyes. On another screen, Dr. Limperopoulos showed me a few graphs pinpointing the location of abnormalities in this baby's brain, based on data collected from hundreds of fetuses. My surgeon's impulse was to find solutions, to fix the trouble spots, but that wasn't the direction things were going in here.

"We're getting there," she said, as if reading my thoughts, without taking her eyes off the image. She said "we," I knew, because her work was increasingly intersecting with discoveries in genetics, molecular biology, and pharmacology. Fetal imaging is laying the foundation for a new era of pediatric medicine. We will soon be starting treatments long before we even thought possible.

For now, Dr. Limperopoulos and her team coordinate their research and findings most closely with Dr. Du Plessis and his neurological clinical team. Imaging specialists are already using the brain database to determine abnormalities in patients on a daily basis and to diagnose a range of fetal conditions. It won't be long before the applications of their work will be more widespread.

During the winter of 2016, the Zika virus was ravaging fetal brains in Brazil and elsewhere in Latin America. Friends asked me if it would be safe to go to Rio to see the Olympics. I had seen a few instances of microcephaly (a small head) before, but the causes were not well understood. I didn't anticipate how soon Zika would be arriving at our own hospital.

At a regular Monday morning meeting that March, Dr. Du Plessis and a team from Johns Hopkins Medicine said they were caring for a woman who had accompanied her husband on a business trip to Central America. She was three months pregnant but had obtained permission from her obstetrician to travel. This was before the Zika virus began dominating the news cycle. After their return to Washington, both the woman and her husband had come down with a nasty cold, but a good infectious disease specialist studying her symptoms—eye pain, rash, muscle pain, and fever lasting for days—identified the culprit quickly. Although this fetus did not have the telltale microcephaly, the mother was referred to Dr. Du Plessis in the Fetal Medicine Institute, where an MRI showed that the dreaded Zika virus had invaded her baby's brain.

The virus's masterful insinuation into fetal brain tissue without revealing its presence for many weeks meant that only highly specialized fetal centers would be able to detect the early signs of fetal brain infection. The mother-to-be decided to terminate the pregnancy and allowed detailed studies to be performed on the tissue, which showed a high concentration of Zika in the brain and in the amniotic fluid. As experts in epidemiology seek to track and forecast Zika's spread to the United States, our multidisciplinary clinic is handling cases from home and abroad.

Severe depression affects hundreds of thousands of pregnant women each year. It has been shown to hinder the development of the fetal brain and have long-term neurodevelopmental effects on the child—effects that may not become apparent for years or even decades.

At the Fetal Medicine Institute, our study of the brains of infants whose mothers suffered from severe depression promises to provide clues to the causes of these ill effects and to address what can be done to avert future problems. Dr. Du Plessis and his team envision a nationwide collaborative approach to fetal imaging, not only to catch Zika but to screen for environmental factors that can affect the fetal brain. They hope to establish a web in which hospitals, pediatricians, and obstetricians have a direct relationship to fetal imaging specialty centers, which are able to process images twenty-four hours a day and screen for markers of conditions ranging from autism to heart lesions. Our dream is for pediatric medicine to begin in utero on a large scale.

This sea change paradoxically means a potential decline of my own area of expertise. The sooner we catch fetal crises, the more successful we will be at eliminating the pain and suffering—and the surgeries—of so many children who are born with genetic and congenital conditions.

A few months before Joe Robert died, he was in his swimming pool shooting baskets with the help of a friend, who would lift him up close to the rim. I was in a deck chair watching and joking. "Someday," he said hoarsely, "someday when I'm not here, I bet you'll be able to catch half these things before the child is even born." After shooting one basket, about two inches from the hoop, his friend gently let him down into the water, and he raised his fist slowly into the air.

That is the abiding image for me as our Fetal Medicine Institute advances in scope and possibilities. Parents today may have a hard time believing what imaging can reveal, but I hope tomorrow's parents will come to expect a precise diagnosis of a range of conditions that can be addressed before they even hear their baby's first cries. We can make these diagnoses in utero now, and clinical trials for interventions and surgeries have already begun: we can now place pacemakers, surgically correct spina bifida, and administer medication to prevent hormone deficiencies. These initial forays into fetal intervention are promising, and they will grow along with our research and imaging potential. This convergence of imaging, genetics, and intervention is one of the most enthralling new frontiers of pediatric medicine.

CHAPTER 28:

Cancer

When I pull my mail from my box at work, I follow a time-tested procedure. I ditch the stuff from pharmaceutical and medical device companies, put the bills and legal documents at the back of the pile, and stack the notes and cards from patients and families on top. Detecting them is easy—a child's handwriting or family address sticker is the telltale sign of such welcome mail.

I open this good stuff first. The letters usually come from current or former patients who are sharing a photograph or description of some milestone in their lives that they might not have reached without our medical intervention. They steel me for the drudgery of the business mail and remind me, while I go through insurance forms and legal documents, that the red tape is well worth it.

One Monday afternoon back in 2002, I spotted a sky-blue envelope in my mailbox and grabbed it. I put it on top of the rest of the mail and carried it all down the hall to my office. I was very tired from a long surgery. My back was yelping at me after I'd spent too many hours on my feet, a more and more frequent side effect of surgery. I needed a boost, and this envelope promised just that.

Using an old letter opener, a family heirloom from my grandfather, I sliced the envelope open with nothing like the care with which I wield a scalpel. Only when it was too late did I realize I was cutting into something inside the envelope—a photograph. I put the letter opener down and finished opening the envelope with my fingers to protect the contents.

The Salt Lake City Olympics were gearing up, and I had read in the papers that the torch runners had passed through Washington. Now I saw that this was a picture of the Olympic torch, carried high and with great pride. I fancied it was a symbol for a patient who had overcome long odds with Olympian courage. I cherished the image for a moment and finally focused on the torchbearer's face. When I recognized him, my heart filled with pride. It was Michael Devaney, that Irish American fighter of a kid, holding up that torch like a champion! I remember his liver and abdomen riddled with rare and deadly cancerous tumors. Michael's parents used to say, "God bless you," with the kind of generosity and conviction that made even me feel their faith. "God bless you," I said to Michael's photograph with a spontaneous laugh.

One summer ten or so years earlier, Michael and his parents had been vacationing in Kiawah Island, South Carolina. At fourteen, he loved basketball. He was playing on a court near their rental condo on a hot afternoon when he took a charge from a boy who was driving for a layup. He fell to the ground in pain. He went straight home, the pain worsened, and then he began vomiting blood. He didn't know it, but a massive tumor on his liver had burst open, and his life hung in the balance. He was rushed to the local hospital and fell into shock during the trip. The hospital resuscitated him, then transferred him to the university hospital in Charleston, where it took a week to stabilize him. The team there did a CT scan and confirmed the ruptured tumor as the cause of bleeding.

A good friend of mine, Dr. Ed Tagge, was a pediatric surgeon at the hospital in Charleston. I'd had several meals with him over the years at conferences and consider relationships like this among pediatric specialists across the country to be key to helping children. He called me about Michael.

Michael needed immediate surgery, and Dr. Tagge told them I had expertise in liver and cancer operations. The family chose to have Michael transferred on an emergency basis to be closer to home in Washington, D.C.

I performed the surgery the day after he arrived. In an operation like this, the general approach is to make a large incision, open the abdomen wide, assess the size and type of the tumor and its position, and ascertain whether the cancer has spread to other organs and tissues. After Michael was asleep, we made the incision, and all of us standing at the OR table saw immediately that his cancer was catastrophic. It was not only in his liver but throughout his abdomen. There were multiple nodules on all the surfaces and linings of his peritoneal cavity and in the intestines and other organs. The liver tumor was quite large, but I had a hunch we would be able to resect the left side of his liver and remove most of it. But the spread of the cancer outside the liver was devastating, and I doubted the oncologists would be able to rein it in with chemotherapy and radiation therapy once we'd solved the tumor crisis. The massive tumor was tricky enough, but the rabid spread of the cancer made me suspect that chemotherapy and radiation would not be effective.

It was deflating to be about to perform a major surgery knowing that it would not solve the problem and would be merely a prelude to another complex intervention. If we were lucky, we could "de-bulk" the cancer, or get out as much as possible to give the oncologists less to treat. But we could not fix Michael by any means, and that bugged me. Our job in the OR was to fix things, and when we couldn't even conceive of fulfilling that goal, our mission took on a different tone.

Before we started, we biopsied the tumor to confirm its type and malignancy. The pathologists quickly delivered bad news—it looked like a hepatocellular carcinoma. This was the worst type of liver cancer—the prognosis was less than 10 percent survival, and that was before considering the fact that the cancer had metastasized to the rest of Michael's abdomen.

I cursed and stood back to reassess what we were up against. I would have to break out of the operating room to inform Michael's parents of the gravity of the situation and to make sure they wanted us to go ahead with an operation that could be futile.

As I emerged from the OR, I realized their son's blood was on my shoe covers, so I slipped them off before turning the corner. As I approached Michael's parents and explained the situation, they did not tear up or tremble for even a second. They stared me straight in the eyes and assured me that they wanted everything possible done for Michael. They told me to proceed with the resection. As I turned to go, out of the corner of my eye I saw them take each other's hands and begin to pray.

I am regularly stunned by the grace of parents under pressure, but this couple had to rank near the top in terms of courageous self-control. They made my spirit wobble for a moment. I walked back into the OR and felt a chill run over my body. A three-minute conversation with this husband and wife had empowered me to regroup. I reported the parents' instructions to the team and told them to get back in there. We were all renewed.

We embarked on an eight-hour operation to remove the large tumor lodged in the left lobe of the liver. To get the bulk of it, we ended up taking out half of Michael's liver. The key was to make sure that the margins of the liver resection were free of disease. We sent the tumor to the pathology department, and while the pathologist inspected it under the microscope, we continued with the surgery, removing as many of the nodules in the lining of the abdomen and other organs as possible. There were dozens of them.

The initial pathology report informed us that we were very close to the margin of the tumor. I felt at this point that we had removed approximately 99 percent of the tumor mass. We had done all we could and had fulfilled our duty—the surgery would allow the boy to put much more of his body's energy into fighting the cancer's source. But that was very different from fixing him, as we would never be able to remove the metastatic and microscopic cancer throughout the abdomen. We were up against a vicious opponent that was almost uniformly fatal. If I could will a cure for anything that kids suffer from, it would be massive invasive cancer like Michael's. I felt ambivalent about cutting out pounds of tissue from a boy who likely wouldn't live half a year.

I closed up the incision and went back out to Michael's parents. It was late in the evening. As I walked out of the OR, I'd never felt more defeated after an operation. I greeted the family, who surely could tell from my demeanor that I was shaken.

"I am pleased that Michael has gotten through the surgery," I began, searching for words to balance reasonable skepticism and hope. "It was a big operation, and we got out ninety-nine percent of the tumor. But I'm concerned about the one percent left behind. The cancer's spread—we got a lot of those nodules, but as surgeons we can't address what we can't see, and I'm certain there's a lot of microscopic malignancy. That said, Michael is young and otherwise very healthy. You've got the bad statistics—we treat kids one by one."

My last line felt like an embarrassing cliché, even though I lived by its code. I always ended with that line about statistics, and usually I believed it. But this time I felt like a damn liar even as I hewed toward pessimism.

"We trust you'll work with us in planning the most aggressive and innovative chemotherapy possible," his father said with total conviction. "He's a very strong boy and an athlete. He's got the fight of the Irish in him. He'll be ready for this."

Michael's parents' serenity was astounding. While they took a walk around the reservoir outside the hospital, I went up to see Michael in the recovery room. As I watched him wink his way out of sleep. I mentally repeated my line about statistics and smiled at him—just as he smiled at me.

Over the coming months, I received updates on Michael's chemotherapy treatments, and each one made me feel an irritating awareness of the limitations of my profession. Our surgery had bought him time, but we had not even come close to giving him his life back. I had worked with oncologists on many cancer cases and had a deep interest in their rapid-fire research and innovations. Their work at the microscopic level was a promising new frontier, way beyond my interventions at the level of organs and tissues. I held out hope that the oncologists could buy him at least a couple more years of life. But I strongly suspected that Michael had come down with cancer about a decade too early to benefit from these innovations.

When I examined Michael a month after surgery, I found his physical recovery nothing short of remarkable. But he was about to go through an amazing amount of chemotherapy, and I doubted his body could withstand it. Like his parents, and perhaps because of them, he exuded an exceptional serenity.

Six months later, even in the midst of intensive chemotherapy, he was back at school. He even tried out for the baseball team with his school's support.

We had confirmed in the meantime that the margins of the tumor did in fact have microscopic cancer, so the only real hope for Michael would be a liver transplant—if the chemotherapy could temporarily wipe out the cancer from the rest of his body. I called one of the top pediatric liver transplant surgeons I knew, Dr. Max Langham at the University of Florida, and he agreed to take the case. The next step, after several rounds of chemotherapy, would be for Dr. Langham to surgically explore Michael's abdomen to assess whether there was still any cancer outside the liver, and to take a look at the edge of the liver to see if there was any visible sign of cancer.

After the surgery down in Florida, Dr. Langham called me. He didn't even say hello. "Kurt, you're just not going to believe this," he said. He could detect absolutely no tumor outside the liver. Nor did he see or feel any tumor along the line of the previous cut. His biopsies showed no tumor, so he decided just to remove several segments of the liver that had partially grown back along the resection line. The incredible findings meant there was no need to proceed with a liver transplant.

Michael came back to Washington for several more rounds of chemotherapy just to finish his treatment protocol, but he seemed to have beaten the daunting odds. Our oncologists and I followed him over the next couple of years to be sure there was no recurrence. Nothing showed up. He went on to have great success in academics and athletics at Gonzaga, then went on to Boston College and later got an MBA at Georgetown.

A few years later on a snowy afternoon, I performed one of Michael's checkups. I had spent the morning operating on Casey, and we were being forced to realize that he would not have the same good fortune as Michael. Seeing them both on the same day, with the striking contrast between their outcomes, only puzzled me. The gnawing question, as I drove home through the snow that night, was why Michael had thrived while Casey was going to die. I was thrilled by Michael's response to an innovative chemotherapy regimen but enraged by the injustice of it all. Michael was lucky; Casey less so.

We are on the verge of transforming pediatric oncology, even more so than adult oncology. The cure rates for pediatric leukemia have moved up to the 90 percent range, and those for pediatric kidney cancer have shown a spectacular rise as well, using a combination of surgery, chemotherapy, and radiation therapy. Bone marrow transplantation, introduced for many types of cancers, seems to improve survival rates even more. But brain tumors and serious abdominal cancers like neuroblastoma are still plaguing far too many children nationwide, and the side effects of the treatment are debilitating thousands of them.

We didn't have the tools to understand the difference between Casey and Michael's responses, but I had a hunch it had something to do with the composition and function of the boys' immune systems. We had helped Michael fight off his cancer, but in the end, his body had taken over and banished it on its own. But we couldn't get Casey to the point where his own cells could do their anticancer work as effectively.

Dr. Tony Sandler doubles as a cancer investigator and was then studying the immune systems of mice. His idea was to exploit the ability of the body's immune system to target a tumor by creating a vaccine from that same tumor tissue. He would extract tumor cells, genetically inactivate them, create a vaccine against the tumor with those inactivated cells, then inject the mouse with the vaccine to stimulate its immune system to attack the tumor.

In lab tests, the destruction of the tumor was significant and, when combined with immune modulators, almost unanimous.

My speech to Michael's parents about statistics and individuals could become a full-blown reality if we could figure how to use the immune system to fight cancer. Immunotherapy was seeing significant success in adult clinical trials, but it was also an incredibly appealing treatment for children. For one thing, it promised to significantly minimize the dreadful side effects of mainline chemotherapy and radiation. For another, while chemotherapy is a wholesale treatment—the same drugs are used across all patients—immunotherapy is tailored to each specific person.

Finally and most important, immunotherapy promised to leverage children's biology in a way that it never could with adults. Children's immune systems lunge for life and healing, just as their bones and organs do. Using immunotherapy, we could harness this unbridled potential and energy—if only the whole medical system, which insists on beginning clinical trials with adults, would let us.

Our success with Michael and our failure with Casey, Victoria's intolerable pain, and Dr. Sandler's work with the immune system spurred me to make immunotherapy our top priority for cancer investment. It felt logical to me because children's biology is programmed to heal and thrive, and because immunotherapy involved so many fewer side effects. Why shouldn't we bet the house on a cancer therapy so perfectly suited to kids?

Joe Robert had taught me that networking and relationships are everything, but sometimes the medical gods bring us gifts of good fortune, too. In an airport in New Zealand, on the way home from a pediatric oncology conference, our head of oncology, Dr. Max Coppes, struck up a conversation with one of the leading immunotherapy researchers in the world, Dr. Catherine Bollard. A native of New Zealand, Dr. Bollard had been at the conference, too. Dr. Coppes began trying to recruit her, and within six months she was heading an immunotherapy lab at Children's National that would soon employ nearly thirty researchers and physicians. Her dream is to make immunotherapy the standard of care for every child with an immune disorder, including cancer. (She and her staff view cancer as just that—a disorder and not a disease.) If their success in the lab and in clinical trials continues, immunotherapy will soon become the baseline treatment at our hospital for conditions ranging from asthma and diabetes to inflammatory bowel disease and food allergies.

In Dr. Bollard's lab, researcher-physicians draw blood from the patient or from an immediate family member and culture their T cells (white blood cells whose job is to fight foreign entities). These cultured T cells are exposed to the cancer cells in vitro, then injected back into the cancer patient. They have been trained to attack only the body's cancerous cells, thereby avoiding most of the noxious side effects of chemotherapy, which wipes out almost everything in its path.

One of the lab's most promising trials is now enrolling children suffering from leukemia. In one recent case, Molly, a nine-year-old with a dreadful cancer history in her family, came to see Dr. Kirsten Williams, a researcher-physician working for Dr. Bollard. A redheaded and freckled spitfire, Molly had undergone two bone marrow transplants with marrow donations from her healthy brother after a heavy course of chemotherapy, but both had failed to kill off the leukemic cells. Dr. Williams's immunotherapy trial was her only hope.

Dr. Williams told Molly during a visit that this time, instead of extracting marrow from her brother's bones, they would take a bunch of T cells from his blood and invite them to spend some time in a petri dish along with what Dr. Williams called a "drill sergeant," a cell loaded with tumor proteins. They would be fed with growth factors and enraged by chemical signals to grow a strong army. The sergeant was going to drill the living daylights out of her brother's T cells, challenging the leukemia-fighting T cells to grow and multiply into an aggressive army. The sergeant would weed out T cells that wouldn't fight the cancer cells, keeping only the strong ones that would dedicate themselves to eradicating the leukemia. The sergeant would then give them marching orders to go into Molly's body and get to work.

"Got it?" Dr. Williams asked.

"Got it, good!" Molly said, nodding up and down.

Dr. Williams infused Molly with her brother's cultured cells on Halloween. The whole time Molly told her how her parents' neighbor's house had a real ghost who was always stealing their keys and locking them out of the house. She was so focused on her story, she barely seemed to notice the blood infusion. Molly's doctors are confident that the immunotherapy will transform her disease into something manageable, if not banish it altogether. Molly didn't even suffer a fever afterward.

Three months into her immunotherapy, Molly has shown an amazing response and she is now in full remission without any evidence of leukemia in her blood. Because Molly had exhausted all other therapeutic options, this cutting-edge therapy was really her last chance, and it has already done more than we had hoped. What's more, Molly's type of therapy promises to diminish or even eliminate unacceptable long-term effects of traditional chemotherapy, including second cancers and heart disease. T cells also offer an important additional benefit to a child's future health: they can persist forever, protecting the child from relapse for life.

The fact that Molly has undergone this trial at all is a minor miracle—due to the structure of clinical trials. The Food and Drug Administration, which regulates medications and devices, requires that drugs be proven safe in adult trials before they can be tested on children. But this is a twofold problem. First, equating cancer in adults and in children is an apples-and-oranges cognitive error. The types of cancer that many adults suffer from (colon, breast, lung) are very different from the most common types in children.

And second, because of their incredibly resilient biology, children may respond better to some drugs than do adults. The FDA nobly wants to protect children from life-threatening therapies, but what happens when a child's disease is already life threatening? As a medical culture, we may be denying these children their last chance at survival. It is a difficult balancing act, to be sure, but as science creates increasingly precise and individualized cancer treatments, the risks are decreasing significantly, and many of the children I have treated would have rushed to be first in line for them.

EPILOGUE:

The Best Man at His Own Wedding

Have you ever sat with someone who you knew was a better person than you? When I was a young doctor and this happened, I would compare myself with my counterpart and set about trying to improve myself in the category—surgical skill, charisma, or humor—in which I felt inferior. Medicine is a competitive world, and doctors can easily get caught up in comparisons of skills and success. I did. But the day I stood in a hospital room signing the discharge papers for a young man named Tyler Williams, I let go of the silly competitive urge that had nagged at me all those years. I knew I would never be a match for Tyler, no matter how hard I tried.

When my colleagues and I talked about Tyler, we often mentioned qualities like integrity, wisdom, and courage. He spent more time asking us about our lives than recounting his own issues; he thought more about his parents' suffering than his own. As a human being, he put me to shame. But I took pride in realizing that along with his mother and father, Nurse Linda, his various other nurses over the course of twenty-two operations, his physical therapists and camp counselors, his grandparents and friends, I had helped forge this young man.

"I want to thank you, Dr. Newman, and your team, for all you have done for me," Tyler said to me that day. "I am sorry to have ruined yet another of your summer vacations."

It had become an August pattern for Tyler to have a crisis with his digestive system, which, over the years, we had essentially built from scratch. His reconstructed intestine had taken hold, but every once in a while—usually a day or two before my family's vacation in August—it wouldn't absorb nutrients properly or would get partially blocked, and the consequent dehydration would trip up Tyler's system. This time his dehydration had been severe, and we had been forced to perform emergency surgery to eliminate the blockage. This sort of blip had seemed to occur every other August for the past ten years.

Tyler's downcast face and regretful voice made me feel guilty about my initial and reliably selfish reaction to his mother's August calls. "Tyler, I'd much rather be standing here signing these papers than burning my bald head on the beach," I said.

"Well, Dr. Newman, now that you can finally go a week late, I hope you wear a hat," he said with a broad smile.

Tyler compelled those around him to stand up straighter and smile a little wider. The kid had survived so much pain and so many scares and close calls, yet with each crisis he grew more resolute about life and human interaction. He reminded me of that Marine in the recruiting commercial on television during football games—as tough and straight as steel.

Three years ago I drove down to a small town on the western shore of Maryland's Chesapeake Bay to attend Tyler's wedding. It was late fall, but the weather was summery, and the light and air conspired to turn my powerful emotions into sentimentality. While I drove, a mental video of my times with Tyler and his parents played on a loop on the road in front of me. I saw him smiling and laughing at his high school graduation party. I remembered the look of joy on his face when he had an uneventful checkup. Absorbed in reverie, I was likely a danger to drivers around me.

As I climbed out of the car in the church parking lot, I couldn't wait for my first glimpse of Tyler's bride, Jessie. In this day and age of superficiality, she must be an amazing person, I thought. Tyler had had a colostomy, colloquially known as a bag, ever since that day I operated on him in front of my wife-to-be. I had often worried about his romantic future, soberly cognizant of the pressures of dating and romance in the digital age. Like a concerned father, I had long hoped he would find a woman to whom he could explain everything he had been through and who would love him all the more for it. At last he had, and I was about to watch her walk down the aisle to become his wife!

I settled into the pew, and the music started. Then Tyler emerged from a door by the altar. In his tux, with his solid carriage and excellent posture, he took command of the room. All the mental videos I had replayed on the car ride down gave way to the powerful reality of this man standing in front of us all. My emotions started in my gut, down in the same spot where I had meddled with Tyler's innards so many times, and rose up to my throat. And then tears streamed down my face.

The organ player began the triumphal march, and Jessie walked in, her father escorting her to the young man who had become almost like a son to me.

I sat back down, as if embarking on a thrilling roller-coaster ride. Throughout the ceremony, I watched Tyler's every move, gesture, and facial expression, at once perfectly timed and genuine. I had participated in this guy's life, I kept marveling. The pride I felt was boundless.

As the minister spoke the names of those we should remember on this day, I thought of Casey, Victoria, and other patients with whom I had developed similarly intense relationships—patients who had not made it. What would I have given to see Casey standing at the altar like that, no doubt cracking jokes during the service? What would I have given to be able to alleviate the pain Victoria had suffered? God bless Tyler, but why couldn't they all turn out this way?

You win some, you lose some. That awful cliché, so loathed by pediatric professionals, popped into my head. I tried to stomp it out of my thoughts. I imagined Casey up there and suddenly wished he and Tyler had met each other. Tyler would have been the perfect dry foil to Casey's garrulous playfulness.

But you know what? I said to myself. The next Casey and the next Tyler are already suffering less and living longer. The children of the generation I have written about in this book, because of their alchemical mix of psychological and physiological strength, of spiritedness and biologic propulsion, have paved the way for the innovations we are realizing at children's hospitals today. Science and technology will improve and prolong the lives of thousands of kids like them in ways we could never have imagined when Tyler was lying in front of me on the OR table over twenty-five years ago.

I watched as Tyler kissed his new wife. After seeing him through so many surgeries and complications, I doubted he would ever be able to have children, but as he and Jessie walked back down the aisle, arm in arm, deeply in love, I knew that that was miracle enough.

Some two years later I had a morning meeting with Dr. Marshall Summar, the head of our genetics lab and one of the leading pediatric researchers in the United States. For some reason I ended up telling him about Tyler's wedding on that fall day in southern Maryland, and I found myself suddenly engaged in a conversation not only about how to make life easier for the next Tyler but about how to eliminate altogether what he had gone through. Dr. Summar's lab was the perfect place to ponder such a possibility. He had participated in the mapping of the human genome and partly because of that work had developed an expertise in identifying and targeting genetic diseases.

Dr. Summar uses precise metrics to identify the seven thousand or so genetic conditions that plague roughly 10 percent of newborns. He aims to tackle them as early as possible, even in the fetal stage, to minimize their effects—or eliminate their effects altogether. He speaks about forever altering adult health through fetal and early genetic intervention.

Dr. Summar shared with me the case of a baby he treated when he worked at Vanderbilt University in Nashville. Mark had been hit with one of the worst possible genetic diseases: carbamoyl phosphate synthetase deficiency. His body could not break down ammonia, a common substance in the body that in excess is poisonous and must be broken down biochemically and flushed out.

Mark's family, who lived in Greenville, South Carolina, scheduled an appointment with Dr. Summar as soon as they found out about his special talents in biochemistry. Little did Dr. Summar know when he took that appointment that they would become neighbors and partners, for Mark's family moved to Nashville to be closer to him. Dr. Summar's work with Mark led to the discovery of the molecular basis for his disease. They became lifelong companions, growing together as doctor, patient, and friends. Mark, now a father himself, still visits Dr. Summar once a year for a checkup, an event that Dr. Summar admits is more a reunion of friends than an examination.

A few days after my meeting with Dr. Summar, I got a call out of the blue from Tyler. It used to be his mother would call me whenever there was a crisis, but he was a grown man now and called me himself. I hadn't heard from him since the wedding, but knew in the back of my head that he would be a lifelong patient.

"Dr. Newman," he began. I couldn't tell from his tone which way this would go. "I hope you are well, sir. How is everything?"

The last time he spoke this way, I had felt an urge to tell him to banish the polite formalities and cut to the chase. But I realized these weren't formalities for Tyler so much as necessities.

I gave him a quick update, and waited.

"I am calling to tell you that Jessie and I are going to have a child," he said. "We weren't really planning on it. I'm in grad school, and we are both working, but we sure are happy about this gift."

I was speechless. I sensed he intuited this, so he continued.

"I asked our doctor if my condition is genetic and might reappear in my child," he said. "But things look good, and he doesn't think our child will run risks that any other child doesn't face."

For some reason, I thought of the towering white cake Tyler's grandmother had made for Alison's and my engagement party—I could taste it still. Then the same overwhelming emotions I had felt on Tyler's wedding day swelled up. So I stuck to the more medical approach.

"Well, Tyler, if your kid ever breaks an arm, you more than anyone know where to come and how to get there!"

We both laughed, and I hung up, still puzzled by the image of that cake. But then I put it together: Tyler's team, both here at the hospital and on the home front, had conspired to give this kid all the help he could ever ask for as he fought his way to a full life. Genetic research, fetal imaging, robotic surgery, and pain research were going to transform the life of the next Tyler, but old-fashioned teamwork would still be the secret sauce for success.

For all the new frontiers we are exploring in pediatric medicine, it will still be parents, nurses, and friends who activate the powerful mix of scientific innovation and children's biology and spirit. I imagined all those people who had sat in the front pews of the church beaming at Tyler's latest miracle of life. Tyler was proving every day Dr. Randolph's age-old lesson that healing children—the fun of it, the challenge, the victory, and the occasional heartbreak—is a team sport, and that the dedication, skill, and passion of every member makes a difference.

Children need to be seen as future adults, and their medical plans require that long-term vision. Their biology is unique, and we should aggressively pursue scientific innovation to give this resilient biology its best shot at thriving. Children's psychology is equally vigorous, and a hospital needs to lay the groundwork for it to flourish. Parents and families are not just emotional bulwarks but medical resources—they need to be empowered as members of the team. Nurses have an important role to play, along with doctors, in executing these objectives, and their leadership role needs to be clarified and encouraged. And pediatric hospitals need to embrace their unique strength as all-kids-all-the-time health care providers. From St. Louis Children's Hospital to Johns Hopkins Children Center in Baltimore, from Seattle Children's to Nationwide Children's Hospital in Columbus, Ohio, the innovations that pediatric research are yielding are stunning but somehow still unheralded and underfunded. This bothers me and I am working with my fellow leaders across the country to make not just pediatric care but pediatric research a higher political and social priority.

If we keep going, and if parents across the country join with us in embracing specialized pediatric care and in demanding its growth and accessibility, young men and women like Tyler will have to learn their lessons in character from places other than the operating room, the recovery room, and the emergency room.

I often lament the heavy use of Latin-based words in medicine because they build barriers between patients and professionals. But these days I tell people that *innovation* has its root in the Latin word *innovare*, "to renew or restore." We are on the frontier of renewing and restoring childhood for thousands of children like Tyler who have been robbed of it by chance or circumstance. That—more than imaging or immunotherapy or robotic engineering—is the ultimate innovation at our fingertips. That is the true frontier. Victoria, Casey, and their compatriots wouldn't have it any other way for the young people who follow in their footsteps.

Acknowledgments

This book started where many end up—in a book club. One of the members of that great group of friends, Greg Jordan, is a writer, and one windy November night in a house overlooking the Chesapeake Bay Greg asked me to share a few stories of the patients who'd affected me the most over the years. I was the chief of surgery at the time, and Greg encouraged me to make notes about these amazing children. Once I became the CEO of Children's National, he helped me turn their stories into a book that could shine a light on the progress we are making in pediatric medicine and the hurdles we still face. Writing these stories and expressing these ideas was as demanding as any intense surgical challenge. As a collaborator and friend, Greg has been with me every step of the way as I wrote this book.

While Greg was helping me, he and his wife, Ali, had their own pediatric crisis. The story of their son Ezekiel and his twin brother, Lukas, became a part of this book. Greg credits the book with saving Ezekiel's life. His experience helped me to understand how important it was to empower parents and give them the tools to know what questions to ask in medical emergencies, and how to access the best possible care for their children.

This book would not have been published without the conviction and loyalty of my incomparable editor, Joy de Menil, who believed in it from the beginning and who provided stellar advice and editing through the various drafts. Joy's assistant, Haley Swanson, was a steadying and reliable quarterback.

My book agents, David Kuhn and the tenacious Lauren Clark, have also been steadfast supporters.

I am also grateful to Gary Marx, my attorney, and to the team at Sterling Foundation Management LLC, who set up a charitable foundation, the Pediatric Health Opportunity Fund, which will receive the proceeds of this book.

The board of directors at Children's National and particularly its chairs, Jim Lintott and Mike Williams, provided vital support and encouragement.

I have had many pediatric role models, beginning with the pediatricians who took care of me in Raleigh, North Carolina, when I was growing up. Medicine is all about education, and mine has been life changing. I worked one summer as an orderly at the University of North Carolina Memorial Hospital when I was an undergraduate at UNC and caught the bug for medicine. Duke University School of Medicine not only saved my life; it also opened many doors for me, especially in the department of surgery. Drs. David Sabiston, Joe Moylan, and Sam Wells were particularly influential. Dr. Howard Filston, the first pediatric surgeon at Duke, provided me with important historical perspective as I was working on this book. The department of pediatrics was inspiring under the leadership of Dr. Sam Katz. Dr. John Snyder was a pediatric resident at Duke when we first met and we became lifelong friends. John and I were reunited at Children's National when I recruited him to become the chief of pediatric gastroenterology. In my last conversation with John, in the summer of 2016, we reminisced about our time together at Duke, which I was reminded of as I was working on this book. He died in a tragic bicycle accident in France soon afterward. Memories of my classmates from the Duke University School of Medicine Class of 1978 filled my head each day as I wrote this book. Many continue to be close friends.

The Brigham and Women's Hospital, one of the premier hospitals in the United States, was a rich environment in which to learn medicine and surgery under the leadership of Dr. John Mannick. I learned so much from its incredible faculty. Surgeons such as Drs. Richard Wilson, Bob Osteen, Roger Christian, and Andy Whittemore were amazing teachers and mentors. The surgery residents I worked with were spectacular and helped convince me that surgery could be an exciting and satisfying adventure. Many of my colleagues in Boston became lifelong friends. Drs. Russell Nauta, Mike Boyajian, and Jay Vacanti were extremely helpful in discussing key details in the early chapters of the book. I will forever be indebted to the Boston Children's Hospital and its medical and administrative leadership. It was a magical hospital for a young doctor when I was training there and continues to deserve its reputation as a world leader among pediatric hospitals.

Several of the surgical fellows with whom I worked at Children's National remain guiding lights, including Bob Connors, Mary Fallat, and Tom Rouse. I was also inspired and challenged by the many other pediatric surgery fellows, residents, and students over the years who made each day in the OR so exciting. I have enjoyed many collegial relationships while serving as a professor of surgery and pediatrics at the George Washington University School of Medicine & Health Sciences for more than thirty years. I had the opportunity to conduct two oral history interviews (with Judson Randolph and Kathy Anderson) for the surgery section of the American Academy of Pediatrics. They were both great friends, inspiring mentors, and incomparable colleagues. Many other colleagues at Children's National provided important details, including Drs. Mark Batshaw, physician in chief, Tomas Silber, and Jim Chamberlain. The CEOs of Children's Hospitals across the country have also been a tremendous source of support, as is Mark Wietecha, the CEO of the Children's Hospital Association.

Medicine depends on the generosity of community members, and so many people have provided key support over the years, helping to fund my vision of what Children's National could be. Fight for Children and its board members were so important to Joe Robert and to me. I am thankful for the leadership there, and particularly to its chair, Raul Fernandez, and its president, Michela English, and now Keith Gordon.

Joe's attorney, David Fensterheim, provided helpful perspectives for this book, as did his family, especially his son, Joseph E. Robert III. Daniel Radek, Joe's former chief of staff, was helpful in reviewing key parts of the manuscript.

The Aspen Institute and its Ideas Festival and Spotlight Health gave me an early opportunity to test out themes and stories.

I am also enormously grateful to the government of Abu Dhabi and the United Arab Emirates—in particular Ambassador Yousef Al Otaiba and the many others in that dynamic country who provided a strong motivation for writing this book.

My executive coach, Susan Kerr, has helped me stay true to my roots and values. As this book developed, I appreciated the critiques of Victoria Dawson and Tom Dann. Victoria was relentless and helped each draft rise to a new level.

My wonderful team at Children's National, and especially my longtime executive assistant, Carol Manning, did so much to make this book possible. Carol has been both a colleague and an inspiration to me for many years. I cannot fully express my gratitude to her. Michelle McGuire, my chief of staff, and the communications team at Children's National, led by Lauren Fisher, and including Rebecca Fried, Amy Goodwin, and Susan Muma, were all fundamental to bringing this book to life. The public relations and marketing team at Viking has also been terrific at helping spread the word. A big thank-you also to Lynn Buckley for her jacket design. Mary Anne Hilliard, chief legal counsel at Children's National, provided sage wisdom and legal advice.

Over the three years of writing this book, the support from my wife and best friend, Alison, from my boys, Robert and Jack, and from my extended family gave me the courage to keep going through the struggles of writing.

Although I singled out one pediatrician, Dr. Ong, to serve as an example for the many pediatricians with whom I have worked over the years, I cannot say enough about the pediatrician for my own children, Dr. Paul Weiner, and his colleagues at the Pediatric Care Center. Dr. Caroline Van Vleck at Spring Valley Pediatrics provided important details about Dr. Ong. I learned so much about pediatric medicine from another great pediatrician, Dr. John

Rusher, during our times together as camp doctors at Camp Sea Gull. There are so many pediatricians who have amazed me with their talent and devotion to children over the years. I also want to dedicate this book to them—they are the frontline providers of pediatric medicine.

My hope for this book is that it elevates the national conversation about the amazing discoveries and innovations we are making in pediatric medicine. Healing children is the first step to healing our society. I thank all the healers of children who have inspired me with their life's work and convinced me by example that medicine is more than a job, it is a calling and a sacred trust.

Eight Ways to Get the Best Medical Care for Your Kids

Over the years I've found myself giving advice to parents about how to tackle the confounding range of decisions involved in finding the right doctors and medical care for their children. A good guiding principle is that the more you use experts and facilities that specialize in pediatric care, the better your child's experience and outcome will be. But there are a few specific things you can do or look for beyond that to become the possible advocate for your child—in sickness and in health.

1. **A few key questions to ask your kids' doctors:**

   For your pediatrician: Will my child see the same doctor or nurse every time we visit? What type of affiliation do you have with the closest children's hospital? Will you refer me there in case of an emergency? Can I call you when my child is hospitalized? Can I put you in touch with my child's surgeon? Is anyone in your practice available in the middle of the night in case of an emergency?

   For your specialist: Do you exclusively care for children? Do you have fellowship training and board certification in your pediatric specialty? For certain issues—namely, concussions, broken bones, dental, and mental health needs—you'll want to be absolutely certain your provider specializes in the care of children.

For your surgical facility: Is anesthesia provided exclusively by a pediatric anesthesiologist? Does the facility have dedicated pediatric nursing? Is a Child Life program available?

2. **Develop an emergency care plan for your child.**

   Childhood injuries are remarkably common—from sports injuries and concussions to broken bones and serious traumas. The best place to take your child in an emergency isn't necessarily the hospital closest to your home. Determine where the nearest *pediatric specialty hospital* is located and find out how it operates. Is it a designated pediatric trauma hospital? Does it have pediatric emergency physicians on call 24/7/365? Are on-call pediatric specialists immediately available? Pick the hospital near you with the most advanced pediatric services and make sure you know how to get there from home, school, sports activities, and anywhere else where your child spends significant time. Map out directions and provide them to the caregivers, guardians, and babysitters.

3. **Find out what child-specific services are covered by your health insurance plan.**

   Is your pediatrician covered? How about other pediatric specialists—particularly ones specializing in mental and behavioral health? Is a pediatric specialty hospital in your network? Will transportation to the closest pediatric specialty center be covered in an emergency situation? These are key questions to ask when choosing coverage, or to evaluate the plan you already have.

4. **Take a tour of the nearest children's hospital *before* you need it.**

   Parents usually don't set foot inside a pediatric hospital until their child is suffering. At that point, dealing with the immediate health issues takes precedence over getting familiar with the people and place that could ultimately save your child's life. Many children's hospitals accommodate general visits. You should schedule one at a time *when your children are healthy.* Take a tour. Meet with nurse navigators, family advocates, and Child Life specialists at the hospital. These are the people you'll want to know in the event of illness or injury. You can also visit the hospital's Web site in advance to understand what resources are available and research the hospital's ratings and accreditations.

5. **Create a plan for specialized newborn care.**

   Expectant moms and dads often plan every aspect of their baby's birth and homecoming but overlook the possibility that their newborn may need access to a neonatal intensive care unit (NICU). The fact is, one in eight newborns spends at least one night in neonatal intensive care. If you are an expecting parent, talk to your obstetrician and pediatrician about referral options for a maternal-fetal specialist. Level IV NICUs offer the most advanced care for sick newborns and immediate access to specialists. Determine what level of NICU is available at your delivery hospital and ask your provider and insurer about transfer options to a higher level NICU in case of complications. Find out ahead of time if pediatric surgeons, anesthesiologists, and radiologists are immediately available in the NICU. No parent wants to think about the prospect of a seriously ill newborn, but being prepared means you can avoid making rushed or uncertain decisions in a time of high stress.

6. **Prioritize your child's mental health.**

   More than 20 percent of children will have a mental health issue at some point in their lives—but parents often don't recognize or admit their child needs help until an average of eight years after the first symptoms—frequently when they have reached a state of crisis. Track and report worrisome changes in your child's behavior to your pediatrician. Find out what psychiatric and social services are available and ask about ways you can take advantage of them. These are important steps that *every* parent should take. All children are subject to mental, social, and behavioral pressures as they develop and grow. Prioritizing mental health is vital not just for kids with established special needs but for *all* children.

7. **Be an active member of your child's care team.**

   At top children's hospitals, parents are considered active members of the care team and their input is *encouraged.* Though the physician is the medical expert, a mother, father, or other guardian can provide details and observations that are fundamental to diagnosis and treatment. This is particularly true for infants, toddlers, and nonverbal children who can't communicate what they feel. When you sense something is wrong with your child but can't put your finger on what, keep track of your observations and share them with your pediatrician. You can also share constructive feedback about your child's care. Most pediatric hospitals collect parent input via standardized surveys. But other verbal, written, and email input is welcome—or at least it should be. In the right hands, a single patient's story (positive or negative) can help spark change across an entire organization.

8. **Bookmark these important online resources:**

For help finding a children's hospital near you: Children's Hospital Association—www.childrenshospitals.org.

To learn more about pediatricians and pediatric specialists: American Academy of Pediatrics—www.healthychildren.org.

To learn more about pediatric surgery: American Pediatric Surgery Association—www.eapsa.org.

To learn about injury prevention: Safe Kids Worldwide—www.safekids.org.

To research hospital ratings and accreditations:

- Hospital safety ratings: Leapfrog—www.leapfroggroup.org.
- Hospital quality and outcomes: Joint Commission—www.jointcommission.org.
- Excellence in patient care: Magnet Status—www.nursecredentialing.org.
- Best children's hospitals national rankings—*U.S. News & World Report*—health.usnews.com/best-hospitals/pediatric-rankings.
- Primary care, patient-centered medical home designations: NCQA (National Committee for Quality Assurance)—www.ncqa.org.

Index